Community and Nurse-Managed Health Centers

Getting Them Started and Keeping Them Going

DEMCO

Community and Nurse-Managed Health Centers

Getting Them Started and Keeping Them Going

Donna L. Torrisi, MSN

Tine Hansen-Turton, MGA

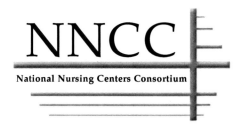

A National Nursing Centers Consortium Guide

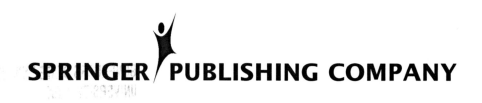

SPRINGER PUBLISHING COMPANY

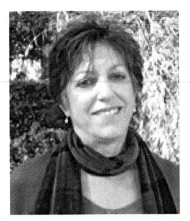

Donna L. Torrisi, MSN, co-wrote, in 1991 a National Bureau of Primary Health Care/Health Resources Service Administration (HRSA) grant to provide health care to residents of public housing. She became the director of this project and opened a nurse-managed health center in the Abbottsford Public Housing Development in Philadelphia in 1992. Since then, her program has received three expansion grants, one in 1994, 2002, and 2003. The health centers are known collectively as The Family Practice & Counseling Network. The sites have been recipients of multiple awards including the HRSA National Models That Work Award and the Smith Kline Beecham Community Impact Award. Ms. Torrisi received the Villanova University Leadership in Nursing Award, the University of Pennsylvania Lillian Brunner Sholstis Award for Excellence in Nursing Practice, the Pennsylvania Nurses Association Leadership Award for Innovative Practice, and the National Alliance for Resident Services in Affordable and Assisted Housing Practitioner of the Year Award.

She was a key leader in the State of Pennsylvania in an effort that culminated in legislative change redefining "primary care provider" to include nurse practitioners. This gave nurse practitioners entrée into managed care as participating providers. She has published and lectured on the nurse-managed model, the art of negotiating with managed care organizations, and on integrating behavioral health and primary care. She is a founding member and the first chairperson of the National Nursing Centers Consortium, and has been a faculty member for the Institute for Health Improvement Depression Collaborative. She is currently completing her final year as a Robert Wood Johnson Executive Nurse Fellow.

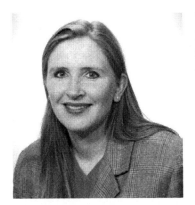

Tine Hansen-Turton, MGA, is currently the Executive Director of the National Nursing Centers Consortium (NNCC), a professional organization that grew from 11 regional health centers to a national representation of over 100 nurse-managed health centers in the U.S. that provide quality primary health care, health promotion and disease prevention services to one million vulnerable families annually. She has a strong policy development background and has been instrumental in changing health policies and regulations at the state and national level, i.e., prescriptive authority and defining nurse practitioners as primary care provides in the law.

Tine Hansen-Turton also teaches health policy, program planning, and outcome evaluation to nursing students in the Public Health Masters Program at La Salle University, School of Nursing, Philadelphia, and is a frequent guest speaker at the Temple University, Jefferson University, and University of Pennsylvania Schools of Nursing, Philadelphia. Prior to joining the NNCC, she was Vice President of Program Development for a geriatric company where she developed, planned, and implemented health care programs for seniors in the Philadelphia region. Earlier, she was the Special Assistant to the Executive Director of the Philadelphia Housing Authority, where she implemented and directed comprehensive health care programs for 100,000 residents.

Tine Hansen-Turton is a member of several organizations, such as the Forum for Executive Women, American and Pennsylvania Public Health Associations, and has published in several journals and books. She is currently President of the National Association of Housing and Redevelopment Officials. Tine Hansen-Turton has published in several journals and is a regular presenter at local, state, and national conferences on health care and housing.

Ms. Hansen-Turton She is a 2005 Eisenhower Fellow and NNCC received a Community Impact Award from GlaxoSmithKline in 2005. She has received several awards such as the State Excellence Award, awarded by the American Academy of Nurse Practitioners 2002, the Champion Award, awarded by the University of Pennsylvania, Health Annex 2002, the Annual Writer's Award, awarded by Center for Mental Health Services, SAMHSA in 2001, and the John Heinz Friend of Nursing, awarded by the Pennsylvania State Nurses Association in 1999. She is currently pursuing a law degree at the James E. Beasley Law School at Temple University.

Copyright © 2005

All rights reserved

Springer Publishing Company, Inc.
11 West 42nd Street
New York, NY 10036

Acquisitions Editor: Ruth Chasek
Production Editor: Janice Stangel
Cover design by Joanne Honigman

05 06 07 08 09 / 5 4 3 2 1

Library of Congress Cataloging-in-Publication Data

Torrisi, Donna L.
   Community and nurse-managed health centers : getting them started and keeping them going / Donna L. Torrisi and Tine Hansen-Turton.
        p. ; cm.
      "A National Nursing Centers Consortium guide."
      Includes bibliographical references and index.
      Summary: "This book provides a step-by-step guide to starting and sustaining a community health center, with an emphasis on nurse-managed centers. The authors share their firsthand knowledge with readers, including information on developing a mission statement, pulling together an advisory board, writing a business plan, and getting funding. The process for obtaining Federally Qualified Health Center Status (and thus federal funding) is described. The Appendix provides examples including sample by-laws, a full policy and procedure manual, physician and nurse practitioner collaborative agreements, job descriptions, a contract with a local agency, and outcome and assessment guidelines" - Provided by the Publisher.
      ISBN 0-8261-2355-4 (softcover)
      1. Community health nursing—United States. 2. Community health nursing—Administration. 3. Community health services—Administration.
   4. Community health services—Business management.
      [DNLM: 1. Community Health Nursing—organization & administration.
   2. Community Health Centers—organization & administration. 3. Medically Underserved Area. 4. Primary Health Care—organization & administration.
   WY 106 T697c 2005] I. Hansen-Turton, Tine. II. Title.
RT98.T677 2005
610.73'43—dc22   2005005646

Printed in the United States of America by Integrated Book Technology.

Contents

To download documents in the appendix and for updated documents, visit www.nncc.us. Click on Health Center Tool Kit, password NNCCtoolkit.

Acknowledgments

Thanks to the many nursing and community leaders who are behind the creation of this manual. Your tireless commitment to ensuring that all people have access to affordable health care is truly inspiring.

This manual is for all of you who struggle to keep your health centers going and for those of you who wish to start a community health center. It is a compilation of much that we have learned in our 12 years of operating and working with nurse-managed health centers nationwide. We sincerely hope that some of the contents will help you in your work. We are grateful to the Robert Wood Johnson Foundation's Executive Nurse Fellowship Program for providing funding that allowed us to create this manual; to Binh Luong, who did a great deal of research and an initial draft; and to Sue Heckrotte for her encouragement and superb grantsmanship that funded one of the first nurse-managed Federally Qualified Health Centers in the country. Thank you to Ann Deinhardt for her painstaking work in editing and assisting with a number of the policies and procedures that are included. Other people who made valuable contributions to the project are Dr. Nancy Rothman, Temple University, Dr. Christina Esperat, Texas Tech, Dr. Bonnie Pilon, Vanderbilt University, Dr. Katherine Kinsey, LaSalle University, Dr. Elaine Tagliareni, Community College of Philadelphia, and Dr. Eunice King, Independence Foundation as well as Family Practice & Counseling's management team who have helped to create many of the documents in the tool kit. They are Dr. Patty Gerrity, Wayne Haney, Kathy Johnson, Mary Moorhead, Peggy Morrison, and Dr. Sarah Rosenbaum.

We are grateful to Susan Sherman, President and CEO of the Independence Foundation, and Judge Phyllis Beck, Board Chair, for being our fortress and continuing to invest energy and resources into our nurse-managed centers and the National Nursing Centers Consortium. We would not be here today without their support and commitment. And lastly, we salute Health Resources Service Administration Bureau of Primary Health Care and Division of Nursing, Resources for Human Development, and all our patients for putting their faith in a different kind of model of care. Thanks to all of you.

Tine Hansen-Turton
Donna Torrisi

CHAPTER 1

Introduction

In the last few decades, the nurse-managed centers of primary health care have emerged as one of the newest innovative models. With managed care systems and state-level reforms being introduced to try to control health care costs, the nursing profession has had increasing opportunities to demonstrate the ability to contribute in the areas of health care access, quality, and cost-effectiveness (Lang et al., 1996). In a landmark randomized control study, Mundinger et al. (2000) found that outcome measures such as satisfaction ratings, health services utilization rates, and health status were comparable between Advanced Practice Nurses, or nurse practitioners, and physicians. Such studies affirm that nurse practitioners can play a vital role in health services in today's environment.

While nurse-managed health centers play a key role in improving the quality of life for many people, they face a number of challenges. Because they are innovative models, they often find obtaining necessary mainstream funding to be problematic. Some nurse-managed centers have had to close due to lack of funding, despite the fact that they have been shown to have a positive impact on the health care delivery system. Other obstacles to sustainability include legal, regulatory, research issues, and problems obtaining third-party reimbursement.

In order for the nurse-managed health center model to continue to flourish, technical support is needed for the development of new centers and the enhancement of the existing ones. This guide has been developed to serve as a resource for people or organizations that are interested in starting new health centers or in learning more about the operation of such centers. It is designed to go beyond the establishment of a health center to address issues of sustainability and questions such as whether to seek accreditation or Federally Qualified Health Center (FQHC) status. The information is organized in a step-by-step format. Within each subject, resources are listed where more detailed information can be accessed. In addition, the guide offers profiles of several nurse-managed health centers in order to provide readers with a glimpse into the operation of various types of centers (see Appendix at the end of this chapter).

THE NATIONAL NURSING CENTERS CONSORTIUM

This manual has been produced by the National Nursing Centers Consortium (NNCC) and the Family Practice & Counseling Network/Resources for Human Development (RHD), Inc. The Consortium was founded in southeastern Pennsylvania in 1996 and has since become a national membership association of nurse-managed health centers. Currently there are NNCC-member nurse-managed health centers throughout the United States, all of which are located in or near medically underserved areas in urban and rural communities.

The *mission* is to strengthen the capacity, growth and development of nurse-managed health centers to provide quality health care services to vulnerable populations and to eliminate health disparities in underserved communities. The *goals* of the Consortium are: to provide national leadership in identifying, tracking, and advising health care policy development; to position nurse-managed health centers as a recognized mainstream health care model; and to foster partnerships with people and groups who share common goals.

The NNCC is an advocate for nurse-managed health centers at the national level. In 2002, the NNCC made strides toward its goal to inform health care policy development and legislative change when the U.S. Senate through a grant to the Centers for Medicaid and Medicare Services commissioned them to conduct a nursing center demonstration project to assess the potential of nurse-managed health centers to serve as an alternative safety-net model for community-based primary health care and health promotion. The demonstration had two objectives: (1) to create an extensive descriptive evaluation of clients served and services provided at 15 primary-care nurse-managed health centers; and (2) to compare select population-based measures of quality and health care resource utilization of nurse-managed health centers to those of like providers, including Community Health Centers. Meeting these objectives answers a specific challenge: to provide documentation of the ability of nurse-managed health centers to serve as core safety-net providers in America's health care system.

Based on the evaluation, the report makes the following conclusions:

1. Nurse-Managed Health Centers are Safety-net Providers
2. Nurse-Managed Health Centers provide a Medical Home for the Underserved
3. Nurse-Managed Health Centers Struggle Financially & Need Cost-Based Reimbursement to be Sustainable
4. Nurse-Managed Health Centers should be Recognized as Safety Net Providers and are viable Partners with the Federal Government to Reduce Health Disparities

Citation: The Nursing Center Model of Health Care for the Underserved: December 2004 Report to the Centers for Medicaid and Medicare Services by Tine Hansen-Turton, Laura Line, Michelle O'Connell, Nancy Rothman, Jennifer Lauby.

On August 26, 2002, in conjunction with the Bureau of Primary Health Care (BPHC) and the National Association of Community Health Centers, the NNCC conducted technical assistance training for NNCC members on the process of obtaining FQHC status. When a health center is deemed a federally qualified health center by the BPHC, the center is entitled to cost-based reimbursement from Medicaid and Medicare, as well as other vital benefits. As a result, the NNCC developed a readiness plan that helps health centers determine whether FQHC or FQHC look-alike status are viable options and whether they are ready to seek such status. The NNCC FQHC Task Force also provides technical assistance through a monthly conference call open to all NNCC members.

To position nurse-managed centers as recognized mainstream health care models, the NNCC conducts over 30 training sessions, workshops, and conferences annually. Among these are the Leadership Program at the Philadelphia Union League and the Annual NNCC Best Practices in Addressing Health Disparities Conference. With the support of the Independence Foundation, the Environmental Protection Agency, and Commerce Bank, the NNCC produced a video promoting the nurse-managed health care model. The video was presented at the 2002 APHA annual meeting. This video is available by contacting the NNCC and can be viewed on the website at www.nncc.us.

The NNCC has formed alliances and partnerships with organizations such as the National Association of Community Health Centers and state Primary Care Associations. The Consortium also works with all of the major nursing organizations to address the issue of sustainability of nurse-managed health centers. The NNCC sits on the Board of Allies Against Asthma Condition, the local and national Lead Alliance, and the National Children's Ten-Year Health Study. For more information, visit the NNCC website at www.nncc.us.

WHAT IS A NURSE-MANAGED HEALTH CENTER?

Nurse-managed health centers are community-based and are managed and staffed by RNs and Advanced Practice Nurses (APNs), such as nurse practitioners who have advanced education and clinical training in a health care specialty. Registered Nurses, Nurse Practitioners and Nurse faculty as well as clinical specialists and Public Health Nurses generally function as the clinical and executive directors of the health centers. These health centers are sometimes known as nursing centers, community nursing centers, wellness centers, or nurse-run clinics. They work in partnership with the communities they serve, often at the invitation of the community, and they are embedded in the core of community life (Hansen-Turton & Kinsey, 2001). Staff includes nurse practitioners, registered nurses, public health nurses, mental health therapists, health educators, community outreach workers, collaborating physicians, and other health care professionals. Although some nurse-managed health centers are located in the suburbs, most serve vulnerable urban or rural populations who would otherwise not have access to health care services.

Nurse-managed health centers are directed by nursed in partnership with the communities that they serve. While today's nurse-managed health centers trace their immediate roots to changes in national health care laws begun in the mid-1960s, the nursing model of holistic care dates as far back as the 1890s. Nurse-managed health centers are usually located in medically underserved areas in urban, rural, and suburban communities. They address health disparities, providing accessible comprehensive primary care and community health programs aimed at health promotion and disease prevention, in addition to behavioral health and home-care services. Nurse-managed health centers focus their care on patients, their families, and their communities (Tine Hansen-Turton, CMS report, 2004).

Health problems or potential health problems are not viewed in isolation, but within the context of societal, environmental, and cultural influences that have impacted the client's past and present health and that have the potential to impact future health. Patients are connected with resources that address and correct the forces that have negatively impacted their health. Providers within nurse-managed centers view their patients as partners in care and strive to provide patients with the knowledge and skills to empower them to assume responsibility for their own health, to make informed decisions about their health, and to become their own advocates. Care is provided by certified registered nurse practitioners (CRNPs), serving as primary care providers, clinical nurse specialists, nurse midwives, registered nurses, health educators, community outreach workers, and collaborating physicians (Tine Hansen-Turton et al., CMS report, 2004).

The NNCC adheres to a modified version of the American Nurses' Association's (ANA) Nursing Centers Task Force definition of nursing centers:

> Organizations that give clients and communities direct access to professional nursing services. Professional nurses in these centers diagnose and treat human responses to actual and potential health problems, and promote health and optimal functioning among target populations and communities. The services provided in these centers are holistic, client-centered, and affordable. Overall accountability and responsibility remain with the nurse executive/director. Nurse-managed health centers are not limited to any particular

organizational configuration. Nurse-managed health centers can be freestanding businesses or may be affiliated with universities or other service institutions like home health agencies and hospitals. The primary characteristic of the organization is responsiveness to the health needs of populations. The nurse is responsible for all patient care and operations (Aydelotte et al., 1987).

While nurse-managed health centers share the core elements of the ANA definition, they vary in their practice models. Services offered at nursing centers range from wellness and health promotion to traditional primary care. Some are for-profit businesses and others are non-profit academic centers developed primarily as student clinical laboratories (Lundeen, 1999). In addition, health centers can be freestanding or sponsored by larger institutions such as hospitals, public health agencies, human services organizations, medical centers, or universities (Riesch, 1992). Centers also vary in methods of reimbursement, which may include any or all of the following: fee for service, sliding fees (usually based on federal poverty guidelines), grant support, third-party payments and cost-based reimbursement available to FQHCs.

The principles that guide nursing practices in health centers date back to the 1890s. Lillian Wald, founder of the Henry Street Settlement for the Poor and Infirm, and Margaret Sanger, who established the nation's first birth control clinic, were visionary nurses of their time. Both were pioneers of the public health movement. Following in their footsteps, the nursing professionals in today's nurse-managed health centers provide health care that is responsive to each community's unique needs.

Today, with burgeoning health care costs and a growing number of uninsured Americans, access to high quality, preventive health care is a key concern for policymakers. Nurse-managed health centers provide a positive solution to the problem. Along with a tradition of community leadership, nurse-managed health centers provide evidence-based care and health care education. NNCC-member centers have demonstrated significant positive health outcomes for patients, including decreased emergency room visits, hospital in-patient stays, and use of specialists, as compared to conventional health care providers. Nurse-managed primary care health centers report excellent pregnancy outcomes, some with close to 100% normal birth-weight infants.

Starting any health care enterprise takes careful consideration and planning. This is particularly true of nurse-managed health centers because they are not in the traditional model. It is suggested that the steps outlined in this guide be taken into consideration by an organization planning a new health center. Those already in existence can also benefit from the experience put forward here.

CHAPTER APPENDIX

Profiles: NNCC-Member Nurse-Managed Health Center Exemplars

The Family Practice & Counseling Network Philadelphia, PA

BEGINNING DEVELOPMENT

In 1991 Donna Torrisi, a Family Nurse Practitioner, co-wrote with Sue Heckrotte a proposal to the Health Resources Service Administration (HRSA) Bureau of Primary Health Care to allow Resources for Human Development (RHD) to provide health care to residents of public housing, under Public Law 101-527, the Disadvantaged Minority Health Improvement Act of 1990. As a result of the grant that was received, Abbottsford Community Health Center opened its doors in 1992 to the residents of Abbottsford Homes and the surrounding community. Abbottsford Homes is a resident-managed public housing development. The Health Center was one of the first seven Section 340a health centers in the country.

A unique aspect of the Abbottsford Health Center is that it is operated in partnership with the Abbottsford Homes Tenant Management Corporation (AHTMC). RHD and AHTMC formed a Health Center Advisory Board, which had seven voting members, four from AHTMC and three from RHD. Among the Board's responsibilities are selection/dismissal authority concerning the health center director, the authority to set policy for the Health Center, and program design assuring that the Health Center programs and operations are responsive to the needs of the community.

Since inception, RHD has opened three expansion sites and has renamed its centers. The Falls Family Practice and Counseling Center opened in 1994; in collaboration with the Drexel University College of Nursing and Health Professions, a second satellite was opened in 2002 in north Philadelphia; and, in July 2003, the Network took over the operation of the Health Annex at Myers in southwest Philadelphia from the University of Pennsylvania

School of Nursing, which had operated the Health Annex since opening it in 1995. In June 2002 the Health Centers became the Family Practice & Counseling Network and the Board expanded to include members from each of the new public housing developments and additional members from the Philadelphia community with expertise that is valuable in the operation of health care services.

MISSION STATEMENT

The Health Centers exist to provide quality, comprehensive health services to all the people they serve with special attention to vulnerable people and residents of public housing communities.

SERVICES

The Network health centers provide a full range of nurse-managed FQHC services to people who are residents of public housing or live in the neighboring communities. Midwives are contracted to provide obstetrical services on-site, as is an integrative bodywork and massage therapist. Some services such as radiology, specialty medical services, and hospitalization are provided by referral to organizations with which the Network has working agreements. In the last year, behavioral health services were expanded at all four centers and a dental clinic opened in the 11th Street Center in the fall of 2004. The primary, prenatal, and behavioral health care services are augmented by health education and support services such as smoking cessation, exercise, and diabetes groups; enabling services such as van transportation and outreach/advocacy; and mentoring groups for youth, such as Teens Making a Difference, Reach Out and Read, and the Peaceful Posse Boys and Girls Groups. The numbers of people served have expanded dramatically to over 6,500. Over the next several years, it is anticipated that the number of users will more than double.

STAFFING

All primary health care is provided by nurse practitioners. Physicians are available for phone consultation and visit the centers about once a month to review complex patients and protocols. Support staff include medical assistants, medical and behavioral health receptionists, administrative assistants, van drivers, and outreach workers who do follow-up with patients in the community and facilitate programs such as substance abuse support groups, asthma safe kids, and lead safe babies. The nurse practitioners also serve as preceptors for primary care nurse practitioner graduate students from several universities and the Network is a site for three or four Americorps members each year.

POPULATION SERVED

The people living in the target areas served by the Network are predominantly African American (88.2% compared to 43% in the whole of Philadelphia) and female (58% compared to 54.8% in Philadelphia), according to the 2000 U.S. Census. The target communities are among the poorest in the city, containing a high percentage of individuals who are unemployed and in poverty. Almost 60% of the individuals in the target communities are under 200% of the federal poverty level, compared to 44% in the city.

Of the people served by Network health centers in 2002, 85.2% were African American and 70.6% of those over 17 were women. A great majority of patients were poor, with more than 80% having incomes under 200% of poverty level. Only 6% had private insurance, 57% had Medicaid, 3% had Medicare, and 32.8% were uninsured.

REIMBURSEMENT

As an FQHC, the Network health centers receive cost-based reimbursement for services under the prospective payment system for Medical Assistance and an augmented rate for Medicare patients. The Network also receives a renewable federal 330 grant and has received federal assistance for several renovation and service expansion projects. Other funds include capitation fees and health insurance payments, a small amount of collected fees and grants from the state and from private foundations.

PARTNERSHIP

The Family Practice and Counseling Network and Drexel formed a unique partnership to extend FQHC benefits to an academically based health center that ordinarily would not have been eligible to be an FQHC. Academic health centers usually survive on temporary grants and are often in danger of extinction due to the lack of sustainable funding. In this partnership, all of the patients from the Drexel University site at 11th Street are patients of the Family Practice & Counseling Network program. The Network is responsible for assuring that all patients receive FQHC services. The Network does not employ Drexel's primary care staff, but contracts with them to provide primary care services. This kind of partnership will support the national agenda to establish 1,200 new community health center access points over the next 5 years.

BARRIERS

One special feature of the Family Practice and Counseling Network is that it is a network of nurse-managed health centers where all of the primary health care is delivered by Certified Registered Nurse Practitioners (CRNPs). The centers contract with collaborating physicians who are available by telephone and they visit the centers about once every 8 weeks to discuss complicated patients. The centers' nurses have had many barriers to overcome, such as acceptance by state regulators and managed care plans to provide primary care, write prescriptions, and obtain medical assistance provider numbers from the Department of Public Welfare, a prerequisite to obtaining managed care contracts. Frequently, managed care organizations allow Nurse Practitioners to care for their Medical Assistance members, but omit those who are commercially insured. With the support of the National Nursing Centers Consortium, legislators, and attorneys, the Network has successfully overcome many of these hurdles. The Network is currently in negotiation with several managed care plans to become participating providers for the plans' commercial products.

ACHIEVEMENTS

Data from one Health Maintenance Organization (HMO) demonstrate the cost-effectiveness of the Network centers. The cost per HMO member for the center was $56.72 compared to $97.96 for the aggregate of all of the family practice providers in the HMO. In addition, clients of the center had fewer inpatient admissions, shorter lengths of stay, and decreased emergency room and prescription drug costs (Kerekes, Jenkins, & Torrisi, 1996). The health centers and their director have been the recipients of many awards, among them the 1996 "Models That Work" award from the U.S. Health Resources and Service Administration and the GlaxoSmithKline Community Health Impact Award.

Most recently, the HRSA Bureau of Primary Health Care cited the Network as a Public Housing Primary Care Model Program. The Network Director, who has directed the program since 1991, received a 3-year Robert Wood Johnson Executive Nurse Fellowship in 2002.

For more information contact:
Donna Torrisi, MSN, Network Executive Director
The Family Practice & Counseling Network
3205 Defense Terrace
Philadelphia, PA 19129
Phone: (215) 843-9720
Fax: (215) 843-7313
donna@rhd.org
http://www.fpcn.us

Temple Health Connection
Philadelphia, PA

BEGINNING DEVELOPMENT

In response to the Nurses' White Paper on Health Care Reform, the nursing faculty of Temple University conducted a feasibility study in north Philadelphia to determine the need for a Nursing Center. They found in that 1992 study that community members were tired of waiting in large impersonal clinics and that over 90% of those who had coverage for primary care did not have a consistent primary care provider.

After submitting a proposal three times, they were successful in securing a 5-year grant from the Division of Nursing, Public Health Service, and opened Temple Health Connection (THC) in 1994. The Health Center operates under the direction of a Community Advisory Board, which is made up of community members representing the Tenant Councils of Norris Homes and Apartments and Fairhill Apartments, the area Home and School Associations, local churches, and social service agencies serving this community. The Advisory Board approves all services and research that takes place through THC.

MISSION STATEMENT

Temple Health Connection is a neighborhood-based primary health care center providing primary care, family planning, disease prevention, and health promotion ser-

vices for an indigent, underserved population at risk, in partnership with the community. The needs of the community direct education, service, and research at THC.

LOCATION

At the same time that THC opened, Temple University adopted Norris Homes and Apartments and a natural partnership was forged between this community, the University, and the health center. Temple Health Connection is located in a two-story corner apartment within Norris Homes and Apartments, which is owned by the Philadelphia Housing Authority and conveniently located behind Temple University Main Campus.

POPULATION SERVED

Temple Health Connection serves the residents of the Norris Homes and Apartments, Fairhill Apartments, and the surrounding community. There are 59,400 people and 12,900 families living within walking distance of the facility. Ninety-five percent of the clients seen are African American and single women head 68% of the families. Unemployment is high, educational levels are low, and close to 50% of the people in the area are living below the federal poverty level. People in this area of Philadelphia live with a number of health problems. The rates of teenage pregnancy, low birth-weight babies, inadequate prenatal care, infant mortality, tuberculosis, sexually transmitted diseases, asthma, and lead poisoning are more that double the rates for the city as a whole. Rates of hypertension, cardiovascular disease, and diabetes are also very high.

In 2002, the THC served 1,686 people in primary care and 3,536 people in disease prevention/ health promotion services. Thirty-seven percent of the people served were uninsured.

SERVICES PROVIDED

The care model at THC is a holistic one, providing a full range of primary care, family planning, disease prevention, and health promotion services.

Public Health programming includes prenatal care, childbirth and parenting education, exercise, weight control and nutrition classes; diabetes and asthma programs; smoking cessation assistance, and additional services such as health fairs, lead poisoning awareness and prevention programs, immunization clinics, and HIV counseling and testing. Community programs include extensive outreach and home visiting, a special cancer program, and after-school, summer camp, and violence prevention programs for children and teens. The students in the College of Health Professions participate in immunization projects, the after school Homework+ program, lead poisoning prevention, anti-tobacco awareness programs, home visitation, and community assessment and analysis. Temple Health Connection is a member of the Nurse-Family Partnership Collaborative where registered nurses visit peri-natal clients consistently over a 2$^1/_2$ year period.

STAFFING

The nursing center is staffed by advanced practice nurses (including Certified Registered Nurse Practitioners and clinical specialists), public health nurses, outreach staff, and office support staff to deliver care in collaboration with a neighborhood family medicine physician. Student, faculty, and community residents volunteer their time for various programs.

BARRIERS

The only barriers are those imposed by a health system that has not yet fully endorsed the advantages of the nursing center model of delivering health care.

FUNDING

The Health Center is funded through third-party payers and contracts, as well as research and demonstration funds from city, state, and federal sources. It has also received funding from foundations, the National Institute for Nursing Research, the Environmental Protection Agency, the Area Health Education Center, the March of Dimes, the American Lung Association, and Temple University Achievements.

Temple Health Connection has forged strong partnerships with the community. Collaborators in providing services include the Philadelphia Housing Authority, Neighborhood Action Bureau, the Philadelphia Parent Child Center, the Village of the Arts and Humanities, the Salvation Army, and the City Health Department Division of Early Childhood, Youth, and Women and its Childhood Lead Poisoning Prevention Program.

In 2000, Temple Health Connection received the HRSA Community Service Excellence Award and the GlaxoSmithKline Company IMPACT Award. The Center was recognized for its work with open airways (an asthma education program) in the schools by the regional American Lung Association. In addition, THC received the National Environmental Education and Training Foundation 1999 National Environmental Education Achievement Award for the National Institute of Nursing Research 4-year funded demonstration/research project, Lead Awareness: North Philly Style, as well as the Commonwealth of Pennsylvania Lead Poisoning Prevention Award in 1997.

For more information contact:
Nancy Rothman, EdD, RN, Director
Temple Health Connection
Temple University, Department of Nursing
3307 North Broad Street, 602-00
Philadelphia, PA 19140
Phone: (215) 707-5436
Fax: (215) 707-3758
nancy.rothman@temple.ed

Texas Tech University School of Nursing: The Wellness Center East Lubbock, TX

BEGINNING DEVELOPMENT

The Wellness Center was started in 1988 by the Texas Tech University School of Nursing and initially operated primarily as a student health service for the Texas Tech University Health Sciences Center in a building on the university campus. In 1998, the School of Nursing decided that, in order to better fulfill its mission to integrate education and service to the community, it needed to change the focus of the services to the provision of primary health care to a medically underserved population. The Wellness Center was relocated to East Lubbock and has become closely imbedded in the community and has been operating there since then.

MISSION

The mission of the Wellness Center is to provide comprehensive health services to residents of East Lubbock, to contribute to the effort to reduce or eliminate health disparities among high risk populations, and to integrate student clinical experience and faculty practice in effective delivery of health care services.

LOCATION

The School of Nursing operates the Wellness Center in Lubbock, Texas. It is located in and serves a geographic area in East Lubbock designated by the Texas Department of Health as both a medically underserved area (MUA) and a health professions shortage area (HPSA). The Wellness Center also operates a Diabetes Education Center in a different area of Lubbock that is accessible to a broader population than that served in the Wellness Center itself. It also has a Senior House Calls program that serves people both in the East Lubbock area and a broader area of the city.

SERVICES PROVIDED

In addition to wellness care and primary health care services, the Wellness Center provides behavioral health care and community outreach, doing both client home visits and marketing activities. The Center provides a practice site for health professions students, and research in the management of chronic disease has become an integral part of its program. Through a contract with the Department of Internal Medicine, screening for colorectal cancer is being added to the services provided. The Wellness Center also provides women's health services to Head Start programs in the city and surrounding towns through a contract with the Lubbock YWCA and Texas HealthSteps services. The American Diabetes Association certified Diabetes Education Center provides education, case management, and supportive services and the Senior House Calls program provides primary care for homebound elderly as well.

In July 2001, the School of Nursing received a $1.7 million grant from the HRSA Division of Nursing to expand services at the health center to include disease management programs for diabetes, obesity, hypertension, and asthma. The Health Sciences Center president added $100,000 to build a management information system capable of obtaining nursing-sensitive data to document client health outcomes. The development of this system has been challenging, but will give the center the capacity to develop credible information about the outcomes it is achieving and provide justification for the need for funding for its services.

STAFFING

The staff of the Wellness Center includes family nurse practitioners, a women's health nurse practitioner, a mental health specialist, a registered dietitian, a clinic manager, receptionist, and a number of student assistants. In addition, the Diabetes Education Center and the Senior House Calls program have a registered nurse case manager/certified diabetes educator, a health education specialist, and several community outreach workers. Currently, the Wellness Center is hiring additional advanced practice nurses to start prenatal care services in collaboration with the School of Medicine's Family Medicine and Community Health department. The overall administrative responsibility for the Wellness Center rests with the Associate Dean for Research and Practice of the School of Nursing.

POPULATION SERVED

The majority of the clients are indigent, unemployed or underemployed, and uninsured. Over 70% are of Hispanic ethnicity and an additional 20% are African American.

BARRIERS

Because its mission focuses primarily on underserved populations and the client base includes a large number of uninsured individuals, a major barrier relative to financial sustainability of the Wellness Center is an unfavorable payer mix. Another problem that this nurse-managed center has encountered is significant difficulty penetrating the managed care market in Lubbock for its primary care services, although the managed care companies are paying for the services of the Diabetes Center and the House Calls program. To be able to move significantly towards sustainability, the health center needs to continue to diversify its funding, including being able to obtain managed care contracts to serve Medicare and commercially insured patients.

Although the Wellness Center provides a full range of primary care services, it has not been able to obtain the FQHC status that would significantly ease the difficulty of financial sustainability. This has been due in large part to the existence of another FQHC in the area that is unwilling to support and work with the Wellness Center in its pursuit of this status, in spite of the fact that there continues to be a great need for the services of both health centers.

ACHIEVEMENTS

The Wellness Center has been able to access significant external funding from public and foundation sources that have permitted the development of additional services and new programs. With funding from the HRSA Division of Nursing, the center has established chronic disease management programs for diabetes, hypertension, asthma, and obesity. Funding from the Catherine and Helen Foundation was used to develop the Senior House Calls program, and a grant from the Centers for Disease Control enabled the Wellness Center to assume management of the Diabetes Education Center. Finally, the center has obtained financial support for a construction project from the City of Lubbock for a new building for the Wellness Center, and will be awarded a grant through appropriations from the U.S. Congress to complete the support for this construction project. The total amount of the construction awards is $1.131 million, and it is expected that the new building will be completed within a year.

For more information contact:
Christina R. Esperat, PhD, RN, APRN, BC, FAAN
Associate Dean for Research and Practice
Texas Tech University School of Nursing
3601 4th Street
MS 6264
Lubbock, TX 79430-6264
Phone: (806) 743-3052
Fax: (806) 743-1622
christina.esperat@ttuhsc.edu

Vine Hill Community Clinic and Vanderbilt University School of Nursing Nashville, TN

BEGINNING DEVELOPMENT

Vanderbilt School of Nursing has engaged in organized faculty practice for more than 10 years. The Vine Hill Community Clinic, established in 1991 with a grant from the W. K. Kellogg Foundation, serves as the cornerstone of the independent, nurse-managed practices. Clinic operations are comprehensive, functioning similarly with regard to clinical services, infrastructure, and accountability, to physician practices at Vanderbilt Medical Center. Since 1991, this faculty practice has expanded to include community mental health, four additional primary care sites, one comprehensive women's health center, and three school clinics.

Vanderbilt School of Nursing has an 8-year history providing preventive and primary care, health education, health promotion, and chronic care management to elementary school students and their families at three sites. Funding from the Division of Nursing in 1995–96 supported the initial clinic at Fall Hamilton Elementary. A second clinic at Stratton Elementary was established in 1997 with partial funding from the Memorial Foundation, a local health care conversion foundation, and the third clinic at Park Avenue Elementary School was begun in 2001 with Division of Nursing funding.

MISSION STATEMENT

The primary mission of the Vanderbilt Faculty Practice Network is to provide accessible, affordable, holistic healthcare to patients across the lifespan with a special focus on vulnerable populations, within a financially sustainable delivery model.

Further, the Vanderbilt Nurse Faculty Practice Network supports health professions education and clinical as well as health services research.

LOCATION

The central (and largest) nurse-managed care clinic in the Vanderbilt Nurse Faculty Practice Network, the Vine Hill Community Clinic, was initially established in Vine Hill Towers (one of the seven HUD public housing project high-rises). Residents and people in the surrounding neighborhoods in this medically underserved area have used the clinic to access primary health care, as well as mental health services and prenatal care. The location of the clinic in the community has decreased transportation barriers to care for residents and given them readily available, open access to their primary care providers. The clinic has produced a rich training site for nurse practitioner graduate students and served as a centerpiece for community health nursing student fieldwork during the Bridge Program (BSN equivalent curriculum). In 2000, the clinic was relocated to the new community center building (occupying the entire second floor) for the Vine Hill housing complex.

STAFFING

Initially, one full-time nurse practitioner faculty member, a medical assistant, and receptionist staffed Vine Hill.

Currently, Vine Hill is staffed by five full-time faculty Family Nurse Practitioners (FNPs), three LPNs, two medical assistants, six clerical personnel, and two coder/billers. With the addition of new primary sites in the past 3 years, an additional three FTE faculty FNPs work across four other sites, as well as 1.5 FTE clinical support personnel.

The West End Women's Health Center (WEWHC), newly opened in 2003, is staffed by four full-time faculty nurse midwives, one faculty women's health nurse practitioner, and three medical assistants cross-trained for registration and scheduling tasks.

1.2 FTE faculty PNP/FNPs and 2.0 FTE registered nurses staff the three School Based Health Program clinics.

POPULATION SERVED

Three TennCare managed care organizations (MCOs) currently assign their enrollees to the Vine Hill clinic where FNPs function as primary care providers (PCPs). In addition, the mental health MCO for TennCare contracts for services with clinic mental health providers. As of December 2002, the primary care center faculty providers were responsible for 7,000 patients under TennCare. In addition, approximately 1,000 commercial and Medicare patients have elected to seek care from Vine Hill nurse faculty providers. Some are members of the Vanderbilt faculty and staff and their dependents. The West End Women's Health Center faculty delivered 340 babies at Vanderbilt Hospital in fiscal year 2003. In addition, these providers serve approximately 100 women's health patients per month. The School Health Clinics serve 1,600 children in elementary schools, with 90% qualifying for the free and reduced lunch program. Primary/episodic care visits to these clinics have generally numbered around 5,000 per year.

SERVICES PROVIDED

Vine Hill Community Clinic and its four satellite sites provide primary care across the lifespan. In addition, community mental health nurse practitioners provide mental health services at the Vine Hill site. Prenatal and women's health services are provided at the WEWHC, and primary and episodic care is provided at the three school clinics.

TRANSITIONS SINCE INCEPTION

In 1994, the state of Tennessee adopted a managed care approach called TennCare as a cost containment strategy. As a result, Vine Hill (and its expansion sites) were incorporated into the TennCare program. The nurse practitioner faculty members have served as PCPs for as many as 9,000 covered lives. The patients often have complex health needs and the nurse practitioner PCPs are recognized as critical safety net providers in the metropolitan Nashville area.

BARRIERS

The greatest challenge is the extremely low reimbursement rate paid for TennCare/Medicaid patients in Tennessee. The per capita expenditures for Medicaid in Tennessee are the lowest in the nation. Vine Hill and the expansion sites face budget shortfalls as a result, while continuing to care for thousands of assigned patients who depend on the clinic for their care.

ACHIEVEMENTS

VHCC and its satellite sites/programs have opened access to quality care for vulnerable populations. PCP visits are encouraged under the client-centered approach employed by the faculty NP providers. Data continue to show higher PCP visits, lower specialist visits, and lower hospitalization rates among patients managed by the faculty nurse practitioners, as compared to patients managed by house staff.

For more information, contact:
Bonnie Pilon, PhD, RN, FAAN
Senior Associate Dean for Practice
Vanderbilt University School of Nursing
210 Godchaux Hall
461 21st Avenue South
Vanderbilt University
Nashville, TN 37240
Phone: 615-322-4340
Fax: 615-343-3327
Bonnie.pilon@vanderbilt.edu

To downlaod documents in the appendix and for updated documents, visit www.nncc.us. Click on Health Center Tool Kit, password NNCCtoolkit.

CHAPTER 2

Organizational Development

CORPORATE STATUS

An initial determination in planning for a nurse-managed or community health center must be whether the center to be developed will operate as an entity under another corporation such as a university, hospital, or another non-profit organization or whether it will be an independent non-profit 501(c)(3) or for-profit corporation. There are a number of options available, depending upon the auspices under which a health center operates. Most nurse-managed health centers today are operated by university Schools of Nursing and have advisory boards to guide their work. In the U.S. centers have the opportunity to obtain Federally Qualified Health Center (FQHC) status under the U.S. Department of Health and Human Services, Health Resources and Services Administration (HRSA), which affords the opportunity for higher reimbursements and federal malpractice insurance. This determination regarding status should be made as quickly as possible. Assistance can be obtained from HRSA staff or the NNCC, which might connect the new center with an experienced Community Health Center or FQHC nearby. New center managers might want to visit both FQHC centers and others, to gain information and explore potential affiliations or partnerships. Assistance may also come from university deans, lawyers, or potential partners such as area hospitals. Filing for non-profit 501(c)(3) status should also be initiated as early as possible. Information can be found at the IRS website, http://www.irs.gov/charities/index.html.

GOVERNING OR ADVISORY BOARD

The Board must be created early in the process of developing the health center, as the Board members are key to the process. The Board may be an advisory board where the center will operate under another organization, or a governing board for independent organizations. Board members may be potential health center users (51% required for FQHC Boards), representatives of health center partners, or experts regarding legal issues, quality of care, or fund raising. A Board should be comprised of dedicated people who are committed to the mission of the health center and willing to work with the management in decision making and problem solving around the development and administration of the organization. Board membership should be such that it represents and is able to serve as a link to the community that the health center serves and reflects the interests and needs of the population. The Board should have a diversity of strengths and capabilities to maximize its effectiveness. It must be determined what kind of skills are needed to start out and what key community figures might be able to help both in the development process and in identifying potential Board members.

A Board must be governed through by-laws, which can be developed using those of another organization as a model and should be reviewed regularly. See Appendix A for a model of Community Health Center Governing Board By-Laws. Minutes of Board and committee meetings should be kept, even during initial planning meetings, distributed to all members, and maintained, organized, and kept as a permanent and up-to-date record, including dates of meetings, names of participants, issues covered, and actions taken. As the organization matures, members of the Board should receive formal orientation to the Board and the fiduciary and other responsibilities of membership, as well as to the organization's mission, history, structure, goals, objectives, methods of operation, and key staff. New members should be provided with a Board Manual and encouraged to become familiar with the health center by means of on-site visits, if they are not users of health center services. Visit the NNCC website for a model Advisory Board Manual (www.nncc.us).

A Board's most important responsibility is the selection and, where necessary, the dismissal of the Executive Director to whom it delegates authority and responsibility for the organization's management and for the implementation of health center policy. This is always part of a governing board's responsibility and sometimes part of that of an advisory board. The roles to be taken by the governing or advisory board need to be decided and spelled out in the by-laws. The Board approves policies that guide the work of the organization and promote sound business practices, quality of services, consistency of performance, and communication of standards and expectations to the staff. It is the responsibility of the Executive Director to assist in the development of these policies and to see that they are carried out. The Board should receive reports from the Executive Director regarding the operation and finances of the center and progress made toward strategic plan goals a minimum of four times a year, and monthly for FQHCs. It is also helpful for the Board to hear regularly from the Clinical Director and other staff and to receive information about the health care environment and marketplace trends.

MISSION

The mission of the organization and of the health center should be determined early in the process, understanding that it might undergo revision over time as the strategic planning process evolves. The mission should articulate the primary goals of the center. The mission should state whether the primary goal is to serve the community and/or to serve as a faculty practice or learning site for students, and whether the center will provide primary health services or health promotion services only. The mission and accompanying vision, principles, and/or values will help guide decision making. The mission statement should be short and clear and should convey the vision of the health center to funders, staff, and patients. For an FQHC, the mission should specifically include the need to provide service to underserved people and to eliminate barriers to access of care. See Appendix B, as well as the profiles of example health centers for sample mission statements.

LICENSURE, ACCREDITATION, AND STATUS

Licensure

A primary responsibility of the organization is to obtain any licenses required for the health care facility; require-

ments vary from state to state. In some states, health centers do not need to apply for licensing, though the facility must be zoned for a health care facility. The center director will need to contact the state's health department or the designated regulatory body for requirements. In addition to licensing the facility, the director of the health center must verify that employees are certified or licensed as necessary. Copies of the nurse practitioners' current certifications and/or state licenses should be on file at the practice, as should a practice agreement with a collaborating physician specifying what the nurse practitioners may do, if required by state regulation. Providers must be credentialed with payers to allow the health center to receive payment for services.

Accreditation

Another issue that needs to be considered is whether the organization will seek accreditation. Among the most prominent accrediting bodies for health care entities is the Joint Commission on Accreditation of Healthcare Organizations (JCAHO). This independent group accredits most types of inpatient and outpatient health care facilities, hospitals and health care networks, and health plans. Although accreditation is voluntary for an organization, the health care industry and the public view this as a "seal of approval" for an organization. Specific guidelines for accreditation can be accessed via the Internet.

FQHCs that do not obtain JCAHO accreditation are approved through a federal Primary Care Effectiveness Review (PCER). This extensive evaluation conducted by the Bureau of Primary Health Care consists of an indepth assessment of primary care services, policies and procedures, governance, and fiscal operations carried out by a team of experts over the course of several days. The team provides a written assessment and a correction plan must be developed by the health center in response to any issues cited and a timeline set for its completion. The PCER process is repeated every 5 years.

Determination of Status

As stated above, there are a number of status options available to nurse-managed and community health centers. Centers can provide full primary care services or focus on health promotion, disease prevention, and education and wellness. Those primary care models that are serving underserved areas and/or populations can also seek FQHC status, but the requirements for such status are stringent and difficult for some centers to meet. The advantages of FQHC status are that FQHCs are eligible to receive cost-based rates for Medicaid and Medicare services and, if they receive a federal health center grant, they are eligible for federal malpractice coverage, saving them a great deal of money every year. The reimbursement rates are calculated based on the cost of services provided in the first 1 or 2 years the center is in operation. The rates are then trended forward based on inflation and are otherwise difficult to change unless new services are offered. Federal malpractice insurance is available to the direct employees of the FQHC and contractors with whom the center contracts directly, rather than through a practice.

Some health centers will not qualify for FQHC status. The most common type of center, the academically based model, which makes up 60% of the members of the NNCC, generally does not qualify. Most of these centers are founded by Schools of Nursing and are operated by the Schools as faculty practices and venues for student learning. Because they are under the auspices of the Schools and/or the universities with which they are affiliated and their director and the staff are employed by the university, these centers have advisory rather than governing boards. These advisory boards generally do not meet FQHC governance requirements, that is, that a minimum of 51% of an organization's governing Board members be health center users and that the Board has control over health center policy and services and the authority to hire and dismiss the director. The same problem often pertains for hospitals and other multi-service corporations that develop health centers. The level of independence and control vested in the health center Board is key to FQHC status.

There are some ways that such organizations may be able to become eligible to be FQHCs. In some cases, waivers from HRSA, allowing health centers operated by other entities to be governed by separate advisory boards which have adequate levels of control, can be obtained where special populations, such as public housing residents, the homeless, or migrant workers, are to be served. Public entities, such as public universities, that meet the FQHC standards other than those regarding governance can apply for FQHC Look-Alike status, which allows them to obtain cost-based reimbursement, but not malpractice insurance. Look-Alike centers can compete for federal grants if they receive a waiver of those requirements. However, a request for such a waiver will likely put the health center at a disadvantage in a highly competitive process unless (a) the request for waiver clearly spells out the authorities that will reside with the advisory board,

and (b) those authorities are substantive, as described above.

Other ways that academic-based centers can position themselves for FQHC status include spinning off independently governed entities and various types of affiliations with FQHCs. Affiliations need to be very carefully considered and health centers are advised to discuss the possibilities in detail with HRSA before taking steps in this direction. Care must be taken to assure that any affiliations allow the center to meet desired goals and do not go against its mission. For instance, affiliation with an FQHC that is not nurse-managed may put the nurse-managed status of the health center in jeopardy. Also, only staff employed directly by an FQHC are covered under federal malpractice insurance; employees of a university working under contract are not. If federal funding is requested for an affiliation to give a health center FQHC status, the proposal must be very carefully written, to assure that reviewers are able to ascertain how the affiliation will work and the way governance issues in particular will be addressed. Several types of affiliation have taken place in Philadelphia and are outlined in the profile of the Family Practice and Counseling Network.

The legislative definition of an FQHC is as follows:

- An entity which is receiving a grant under Section 329, 330, 340, or 340a of the Public Health Service (PHS) Act;
- An entity which is receiving funding from such a grant under a contract with the, grantee and which meets the requirements to receive a grant under Section 329, 330, 340, or 340a of the PHS Act;
- An entity that, based on the recommendation of the Health Resources and Services Administration (HRSA), is determined by the Secretary to meet the requirements for receiving a grant under Section 329, 330, 340, or 340a of the PHS Act;
- An entity receiving grant funds either directly or indirectly is defined by the scope of the approved Section 329, 330, 340, or 340a grant application with respect to size, organizational structure, and location of the facility or facilities;
- An outpatient health program or facility operated by an Indian tribe or tribal organizations under the Indian Self-Determination Act (Public Law 93-638);
- An Urban Indian organization receiving funds under Title V of the Indian Health Care Improvement Act for the provision of primary health services;
- An entity which was treated by the Secretary for purposes of Part B of Title XVII as a comprehen-

sive federally funded health center as of January 1, 1990.

Federally Qualified Health Centers must meet standards in a number of areas.

- Need and Community Impact

  - Demonstrate the need for services in the community based on geographic, economic, and demographic factors; other area resources; and health status of the population.
  - Applicant must serve those most in need within the service area, including low-income individuals, the uninsured, minorities, pregnant women, the elderly, migrant or seasonal farmworkers, and, where appropriate, those with special needs.
  - Must serve a designated Medically Underserved Area (MUA) or Medically Underserved Population (MUP).

- Health Services

  - Applicant must provide the following services, either directly, through contract, or through formal referral arrangements with accountability to the applicant: primary health care services by physicians, nurse practitioners, physician assistants; diagnostic laboratory services; diagnostic x-ray services; patient case management; pharmacy services needed to complete treatment; mental health services, prenatal care, preventive dental services; emergency services; and transportation for patients who would otherwise lack access services.
  - All contracted services must remain under the governance, administration, clinical management, and quality assurance (including record review) of the applicant organization. This will be affirmed through a description of accountability for all contracted services and submission and review of contract documents for any contracted services comprising more than 10% of costs submitted by the entity for payment.
  - The applicant must ensure full representation of the target population in receiving FQHC services (i.e., the population served may not be limited by age or gender). This requirement may be achieved through the prime contractor or a network arrangement that meets the contracting requirements described above.

- Applicant must demonstrate that it maintains a core staff of full-time primary care providers (i.e. physicians and nurse practitioners, physician assistants, certified nurse midwives).
- Applicant must demonstrate that there is a sufficient but not excessive number of primary care providers in relation to the persons served.
- All primary care providers, with the exception of certain National Health Service Corps providers, are licensed to practice in the State where the center is located.
- Applicant's primary care providers have hospital admitting privileges or, in cases where this is not feasible, the applicant must have referral arrangements in place for hospitalization and discharge planning, which ensures continuity of care.
- Services must be available to all, regardless of ability to pay.
- The applicant must use a charge schedule with a corresponding discount schedule based on income.
- The applicant must be open at least 32 hours per week, providing services at times that meet the needs of the majority of potential users. Applicant should indicate whether early morning, evening, or weekend hours are scheduled each week.
- The applicant must provide professional coverage during hours when the center is closed. The applicant must demonstrate firm arrangements for after-hours coverage by their own providers and, if necessary, other community providers. This system must ensure telephone access to a health care provider who is part of the center's after-hours system.
- The applicant must have an ongoing quality improvement program that identifies problems and allows for necessary actions to remedy problems.

- Management and Finance

  - The applicant's organization should have a line of authority from the Board to a chief executive (President, CEO, or Executive Director) who delegates, as appropriate, to other management and professional staff, including a Finance Director and a Clinical and/or Medical Director. An organizational chart reflecting these positions and their relationships should be maintained and periodically updated by the chief executive and provided to the Board.

- The applicant must have systems which accurately collect and organize data for reporting and which support management decision making. The applicant must be able to integrate clinical, utilization, and financial information to reflect the operations and status of the organization as a whole.
- The applicant must have accounting and internal control systems appropriate to the size and complexity of the organization.
- The applicant must have in place written billing, credit, and collection policies and procedures, including a system for billing patients and third parties within 45 days of a service being rendered; a procedure for aging accounts receivable, producing appropriate aging reports, and following up on overdue accounts to ensure collection; and a procedure for handling bad debts on a regular basis.
- The applicant must demonstrate that an annual independent financial audit is performed in accordance with federal audit requirements.
- If problems are cited in the audit or report on internal controls, these problems must be explained and adequate procedures must be in place to correct those problems.
- The applicant must demonstrate that annual revenues equal 90% of expenditures. Revenues and expenditures are to be reported upon application and substantiated by the audit.
- The applicant must demonstrate that it has, or has applied for, a Medicaid provider number as an FQHC.
- The applicant must demonstrate that it is a Medicare provider if serving patients over 65 or SSI patients.

- Governance
  - The applicant must be a public or private non-profit entity as certified through Federal or state process.
  - The applicant's governing board must have 9 to 25 members, the majority (at least 51%) of whom are active users of the center and who, together, represent the user population of the center. The board is expected to meet monthly. In the case where the governing board is a university or other corporation serving a broader range of constituents, an Advisory Board that consists of a minimum of 51% health center users may govern the health center. In this case, the governing board will not have a majority of health center users and a waiver may be obtained from the federal government. Waivers from monthly meetings may also be requested. No more than half of the non-user governing board members may derive 10% or more of their income from the health care industry.
  - If the applicant is a private, non-profit organization, the governing board must have full authority and responsibility for center operations. Specifically, the governing board must have the authority to approve the center's budget, approve the selection and dismissal of the top-level management, and set center policies.
  - If the applicant is a public entity, the governing board must have the same authority as the governing board of a private, non-profit organization, except that the public agency may retain the authority to establish general (fiscal and personnel) policies for the center. There must be a written agreement between the governing board and the public agency delineating the roles and responsibilities of each entity. The governing board must have the authority to approve the center's budget, approve the selection and dismissal of the top-level management, and set center policies.
  - The by-laws or written corporate policies of the applicant must include provisions that prohibit conflict of interest or the appearance of conflict of interest by board members, employees, consultants, and those who provide services or furnish goods to the applicant. No board member may be an employee of the center or be an immediate family member of an employee.

FQHC standards are based in sound practice. Those standards, other than the specifics regarding governance, have been used in the development of this guide. Links to FQHC information are available on the National Nursing Centers Consortium website at http://www.nncc.us.

Resources for Licensure and Accreditation:

Buppert, C. (1999). *Nurse practitioner's business practice and legal guide.* Gaithersburg, MD. Aspen Publication, Inc.

Bureau of Primary Health Care website: http://bphc.hrsa.gov

Joint Commission on Accreditation of Healthcare Organizations website: http://www.jcaho.org

National Council of State Boards of Nursing website: http://www.ncsbn.org

SITE SELECTION

Selecting the site for a health center requires significant study and planning. It is imperative that the center be located in an area where there is a defined need not being met by any other provider(s). This is especially necessary for a center seeking federal funding or FQHC status, since the government, like most funders, does not want to fund duplicate services. Geographic accessibility for the target population, including ease of public transportation and parking, is a key consideration. The financial resources available will dictate whether the facility should be rented or purchased. The services to be provided at the health center will determine the size and layout of the physical space.

The specific population to be served may also affect site selection. For instance, the Family Practice & Counseling Network serves public housing residents and works in collaboration with the Philadelphia Housing Authority; thus all sites are located in or near public housing developments. Other NNCC member health centers are located in churches, community and recreation centers, and shopping malls.

Zoning is another factor in site selection. Zoning is the way government controls the physical development of land and uses of property. Even though a space may have commercial zoning, it is important to know whether or not it can be utilized as a health center. Depending on the local rules and ordinances, some businesses will need a permit or license to operate. An organization would do well to contact local political entities and/or a lawyer early in the process to assure that sites being considered are viable possibilities.

Resources for site selection:

Free Advice on Zoning: http://real-estate-law.freeadvice.com/zoning

Free Advice on State Laws: http://law.freeadvice.com/resources/statecodes.htm

U.S. Chamber of Commerce website: http://www.uschamber.com

CHAPTER 3

Initial Planning

Once a determination has been made as to the type of health center that will be operated and the initial board has been formed, the formal planning for the health center can begin. Sometimes some of the needs assessment will be done before these determinations are made.

NEEDS ASSESSMENT

Since nurse-managed and community health centers are community focused, a comprehensive, written community needs assessment should be done to assure that the programs and services that are developed are as responsive as possible to the community. It will be important to identify the population to be served; the beliefs, values, and attitudes of the community; and the barriers that exist in the community to quality health care. Assessing the community will provide health care professionals with an understanding of community dynamics and how they contribute to or detract from the state of health of the population (Clemen-Stone, McGuire, & Eigsti, 2002). The assessment may also help to identify the unmet needs of the population and the health disparities between it and the larger community, as well as avoid duplication of services. This type of community needs assessment should be ongoing, because communities are dynamic systems and continuing changes will affect the need for services (Lundeen, 1999).

The focus of the needs assessment should be on the community's strengths and existing resources. Any community organizations that have similar interests and may be potential collaborators or competitors should be identified and studied. This type of review can reduce the chance of duplication of services and could lead to a comprehensive array of services through collaboration, resource sharing, and cost effectiveness. Other benefits of collaboration or affiliation may be the promotion of

commitment to community health improvement efforts, the activation of citizens to participate in health decision making, and the promotion of a shared vision regarding community health goals and outcomes (Clemen-Stone et al., 2002).

Community assessments should have a variety of components. Analyzing data that is descriptive of the geographic area and the population and any sub-populations to be served, such as census data, local health status data, and vital statistics, is one important way of assessing the needs of the target group. Data could include age, sex, socioeconomic status, ethnicity/culture, language, HIV prevalence, and health disparities when comparisons are made with a larger population. It is important to determine the community's status as a Medically Underserved Area (MUA) or Medically Underserved Population (MUP) and to compare local statistical information to national data, including those available on the Centers for Disease Control (CDC) Website, and *Healthy People 2010* data, which can be found on http://www.healthypeople.gov. Sociodemographic characteristics of the area can be obtained from state and federal agencies. These qualitative and quantitative data help identify at-risk populations and specific high-priority health issues.

Local organizations and community leaders are invaluable resources because of their links to the community. Utilizing them in the development of a health center will help to identify gaps in health care services and ensure that the health care programs developed are suitable to the culture of the community. There are several means to assess community information, including face-to-face interviews with community residents and leaders, town hall meetings, and review of community newspapers and organization publications. In addition, organization staff can conduct neighborhood windshield surveys and walking tours; that is, tours of a geographic area at varying times to observe and record information and community characteristics (Clemen-Stone et al., 2002).

According to Glick, Hale, Kulbok, and Shettig (1996), the success of a community-based program is dependent upon community member participation and the fostering of a sense of neighborhood "ownership." It is vital that some of the methods noted above are used to ensure that, from the outset, the community is aware of the plans being made by the organization, community leaders have real input in the development process, and services provided by the health center are culturally appropriate and accessible to the target population. Community input should not be limited to the needs assessment and planning process.

The Family Practice & Counseling Network, a network of nurse-managed FQHC primary care centers in Philadelphia, is an example of an organization that has an ongoing collaborative effort with community residents. It is one of the example organizations profiled later in this manual. The Network centers serve several public housing developments and empower the communities served by operating with a tenant-driven Advisory Board that has representation from all of the communities served. The Board hires the Director and delegates to that person the management responsibility for the center, including all responsibility for selection and dismissal of staff. The Board also approves the Network's budget, major policies, and strategic plan, as well as all grant applications and decisions regarding additions of sites or services.

An organization coming into an underserved community should expect that initially community members might be reluctant to trust. This is not surprising given their history of use, abuse, and broken promises. It is imperative that nursing leaders be sensitive to this and willing to work through these difficult issues in order to establish a lasting and trusting partnership. Open dialogue between the organization and community residents can help build rapport and trust and is critical to the development of services that are culturally appropriate and community focused.

STRATEGIC PLANNING

An organization that is planning to develop a health center should first create a comprehensive, written strategic plan that covers a 2 to 5 year period and includes a long-range financial plan and a capital plan to accomplish determined goals. The strategic plan must have input from the Board, staff, and community leaders and should be approved by the Board. See Appendix C for a model strategic planning policy and procedure.

An internal assessment should be done that includes a SWOT (Strengths, Weaknesses, Opportunities, and Threats) analysis and considers the organization's resources and staff skills, as well as its limitations. Analysis should consider reimbursement trends and the center's competitive position and should include the following: (a) existing services, (b) services restricted by third-party payers, (c) services expanded to meet third-party requirements, and (d) potential services that provide more comprehensive care (Kinsey & Gerrity, 1997). The Board and management should review and either affirm or revise the mission of the organization.

The strategic planning effort should use the information from the community assessment, as well as the internal assessment or strategic analysis, to develop a comprehensive plan for services to be provided, collaborations/affiliations to be established, and a financial plan and capital plan that take into account all pertinent issues. The range of services that will be provided, either directly or indirectly, should be specified. The number of practitioners and support staff needed to operate should be detailed, as well as their required credentials. The center's need for volunteers and the ways they can be recruited, used, and monitored should also be considered. The mechanisms for including the community in the planning and management of the center and its services should be part of the plan, as should the center's plan for participating in the community and local, state, and national networks. A model Strategic Plan is included in Appendix D.

Resources for Strategic Planning:

Strategic Planning Consultants:
    Ann Deinhardt—acdeinhardt@comcast.net;
    Dyann Mowatt Roth—DyMowatt@msn.com;
    Ellen Tichenor—Tichassociates@aol.com
Clarkston Health Collaborative—Windshield Survey: http://mapp.naccho.org/ctsa/CtsaClarkstonWindshieldSurvey.asp
Community Health Data Base: http://www.phmc.org/chdb
Conducting a Community Assessment: http://www.ncrel.org/sdrs/areas/issues/envrnmnt/css/ppt/chap2.htm
Healthy People 2010 website: http://www.healthypeople.gov
Kriegler, N., & Harton, M. (1992). Community health assessment tool: A patterns approach to data collection and diagnosis. *Journal of Community Health Nursing, 9*(4), 229–234.

National Center for Health Statistics: http://www.cdc.gov/nchs/nvss.htm

National Network for Health website: http://www.nnh.org

National Nursing Centers Consortium: http://www.nncc.us

Neuber, K. A. (1980). *Needs assessment: A model for community planning*. Newbury Park, NJ: Sage Publications.

Rissel, C., & Bracht, N. (1999). Assessing community needs, resources, and readiness: Building on strengths. In N. Bracht (Ed.), *Health promotion at the community level: New advances* (2nd ed., pp. 59–71). Thousand Oaks, CA: Sage.

Strategic Planning in Smaller Nonprofit Organizations: http://www.wmich.edu/nonprofit/guide7.htm

U.S. Census Bureau—American Community Survey: http://www.census.gov/acs/www/Products/Profiles/index.htm

TABLE 3.1 Start-Up Checklist

Checklist	Questions to Think About	Advice from Experts
Getting 501c3 Status	Will the health center be an independent 501c3 or will it operate under the umbrella of another non-profit entity?	• Having its own 501c3 status allows a center greater financial freedom and the opportunity to obtain FQHC status. Information on the process of filing for 501c3 status can be found at the IRS Website http://www.irs.gov/charities/index.html
Create a Governing or Advisory Board	What kind of skills do you need to start out? Whom do you know who has these skills? What key community figures might be able to help?	• A board should be comprised of a group of dedicated people to share tasks and problem solve. Health center users are required to comprise a minimum of 51% of the board in an FQHC. In addition to health center users, board members may be health center partners or people who are experts at fund raising, legal issues, and quality of care. • Find others in the community doing similar work and utilize them as resources. A sample of Community Health Center governing board by-laws is in Appendix A. Job descriptions should reflect the mission (see Appendix N)
Mission Statement	What is the primary goal of the health center? What is the guiding principle behind starting the health center?	• The mission helps guide decision making and articulate the vision of the health center to funders, staff, and patients. • Keep it short and clear. It should reflect the long-term vision for the health center.
Needs Assessment	Who in the community will be the target population? What is the population profile of the community? What is the status of the existing health care delivery system? What will be the range of services for the health center?	• Start with existing data such as the U.S. Census data, local health department, local United Way, or local hospital statistics to gain a better understanding of the needs of the community.
Rules and Regulations	What are the state, city, and local laws that pertain?	• Being well informed about rules and regulations will help prevent malpractice and other legal problems.
Resource Assessment	What services are other agencies in the area providing? Are there any gaps in the service? What are the eligibility requirements for Medicare and Medicaid?	• This will help determine the types of services the health center should offer and will help identify potential partnerships and referral sources.
Financial	How much money is needed to start the health center? How and where will the center seek donations and grants? How will the billing system work?	• This will guide the services that will be provided by the health center and will help identify gaps.
Insurance	What type of insurance will the center need? What type of liability coverage will the practitioners need?	• There are two types of liability coverage: professional liability insurance for the provider and comprehensive general liability policy for the facility. • Under the Federally Supported Health Centers Assistance Act, health centers funded under section 330 of the Public Health Service Act are eligible for medical malpractice insurance program at no cost to the grantee (Federal Tort Claim Act). • Other health centers will need to purchase private professional liability insurance. Requirements vary state-to-state. See http://www.hpso.com

(continued)

TABLE 3.1 *(continued)*

Checklist	Questions to Think About	Advice from Experts
Space and Site Selection	Is the location in a Medically Underserved Area (MUA), a Health Professional Shortage Area (HPSA), or in an area with a special medically underserved population? Where should the center be located to be most accessible to the target population? How many rooms and offices are needed? Is a conference room necessary?	• It is key to locate services in an area of need and to avoid duplication of existing services. Duplication will handicap the center's ability to receive grants and FQHC status. • Take into consideration the number of clients to be served, how much space is needed for exam or meeting rooms and offices, and accessibility by public transportation. • Generally one primary care clinician needs a minimum of two exam rooms to maximize productivity.
Staffing	How many practitioners and support staff does the health center need to operate? Does the center need volunteers and how will they be recruited? What credentials are required?	• Generally a ratio of two to three support staff (MA, RN or LPN, Front Desk) per full time clinician will allow the generation of 16–22 patients a day.
Business Operations	What hours of operation are needed? What type of call system will be set up to ensure that patients have 24-hour access to providers, where necessary?	• What are State regulations re: payers contracting with independent Nurse Practitioners? • Expectations for an FQHC are a minimum of 20 hours per week, 52 weeks a year. • 24-hour telephone on-call is required for primary care.
Licenses and Approvals	Is all the necessary paperwork completed to comply with relevant state and federal requirements? What equipment is needed? Is a laboratory needed?	• The state and federal governments must approve even practices with a small lab. A CLIA (Clinical Laboratory Improvements Amendments) certification is required for all labs. A lab limited to performing "waived" tests is subject to less regulation. Waived tests include but are not limited to hct or hgb, urine dipstick, urine pregnancy test, fingerstick blood sugars and hemocult, and vaginal wet smears. Waived tests may vary; regulations may change as new reliable tests become available. See http://www.cms.hhs.gov/clia
Credentialing, Quality Improvement/Quality Assurance	What is the credentialing process in the particular service area? How will the center measure the quality of care that the patients receive?	• APNs must have proper certification. This is essential to be credentialed by managed care organizations and impacts the prevention of successful malpractice suits. All primary care, behavioral health, and specialty providers must be credentialed. It is advisable that a National Data Bank Search be conducted. (See Appendix J for a sample credentialing procedure) • A system must be in place to maintain quality of care for patients and the management of the health center. A Quality Improvement Committee should be established. • The NNCC Quality Management Document is a helpful resource and is available on the NNCC website.

CHAPTER 4

Ongoing Planning

The strategic planning process should be completed at least once every 2 to 5 years. For FQHCs, the process must be completed at least every 3 years, before the project period grant submission, and must be reviewed formally every year. Each year, annual plans should be developed, including both program and business strategies, that support the goals of the strategic plan and allow for changes in strategies as the environment and internal processes of the health center change. For FQHCs, these annual plans are developed in Health Care Plan and Business Plan formats that are required by HRSA. These formats can enhance the strategic planning process for all health centers, however. The Executive Director should make periodic reports to the Board regarding progress made toward implementation of the strategic plan, the annual health care and business plans, and the annual and capital budgets, and she should make recommendations for changes as necessary.

The Health Care Plan is a concrete plan that sets specific clinical service goals and describes specific actions to be taken over the coming year to maintain and/or improve quality of care and outcomes. The Health Care Plan should focus on the highest priority needs and health disparities of the population and should support and be congruent with the Strategic Plan. It should be the working document for the health center staff for the year.

The Health Care Plan usually follows the life cycles and addresses the following:

- Maternal health;
- Infant, pediatric, and adolescent health;
- Men's and women's issues;
- Geriatric services;
- Oral health; and
- Chronic illness.

If behavioral health or other clinical services are provided, these should also be included. The Health Care Plan should include a review of progress toward goals set in the strategic plan.

The individuals in the organization with clinical expertise in primary care and behavioral and oral health write the Health Care Plan, if these services are provided. Getting as many clinicians as feasible to help write the plan helps promote buy-in, engagement, and a quality document. It is important that all staff are aware of the content of the Plan. The Board must approve the Plan.

The components of the Health Care Plan can vary. The Bureau of Primary Health Care has a format for section 330 funded programs that include the following sections:

- Achievable, Time-framed, and Measurable Goals and Objectives,
- Key Action Steps,
- Data Sources and Evaluation Methods,
- Outcomes and Indicators and Measurements of Success,
- Person/Area Responsible, and
- Progress Made/Comments.

Benchmarks for success should be set for each goal in a Health Care Plan. Health Employment Data Information Set (HEDIS) measures and Healthy People 2010 goals may serve as benchmarks. Whenever possible, the goals set in the Health Care Plan should reach or exceed HEDIS or Healthy People goals. Progress toward Health Care Plan goals should be monitored through the organization's Quality Improvement process. See Appendix E for a sample health care plan.

A Business Plan covers the financial and other goals of the organization and complements the Health Care Plan. The steps below can assist in the development of both the Health Care Plan and the Business Plan for the organization.

- Begin by gathering quality improvement information, market research information, and financial information that will help to develop and support the strategic plan.
- Set concrete, measurable goals and objectives that support the goals of the long-term strategic plan. An example goal might be: In the next twelve months, the number of health center users will increase by 500 people.
- Based on the objectives listed, an outline of a concrete strategy or key action steps for achieving them should be developed. An example of a strategy might be: The health center will contract with the Haven Homeless Shelter to be the primary health care provider for their 300 residents.
- The person or unit responsible for each step should be specified. A plan is only as good as the people who will make it happen. Note who is responsible for each key action step and be clear about the timeframe in which each step is to be accomplished.
- A financial plan to support the plans should be developed to be sure of their feasibility.
- Prepare an Executive Summary that summarizes the ideas that are developed in the plan. The purpose of an Executive Summary is to leave the reader with a concise, convincing statement of the plan and its feasibility.

Particularly for the initial plans, the organization should identify people with background knowledge of the planning process, health center management, and business management to review the Health Care and Business Plans for completeness, logic, efficacy as a communication and management tool, and presentation.

Business Plans are covered in chapter 5.

CHAPTER 5

Funding

There are a number of funding options for health centers, including federal, state, local, and private grants, state and local contracts, third-party reimbursement, and fee-for-service. There are advantages and disadvantages to each option. Because there is not a single model to depend on in establishing a viable financial base, it is important for nurse-managed health centers to cultivate multiple funding streams to support the best possible cash flow. Most nurse-managed centers are supported by a patchwork of public and private funding sources. The financial development process requires a great deal of flexibility and creativity.

FEDERAL, STATE, AND LOCAL GRANTS

Obtaining a major grant can secure the finances of a health center for the length of the grant. Such funding can enhance the health center's public image and may leverage other funding as well. If a health center qualifies as a FQHC, it can receive ongoing funding through the HRSA Community Health Care funding stream. Other time-limited funding includes HRSA, Division of Nursing funding.

If it is an option and a health center has a significant number of Medicare or Medical Assistance clients, FQHC status can assure cost-based reimbursement for Medical Assistance primary care visits and an augmented rate for Medicare. This can make the difference between a capitation rate of $9.00 per member per month and a per-visit reimbursement rate of $120 per visit, depending on the center's actual cost per visit. HRSA also provides opportunities for FQHC centers to obtain funding that will allow for service expansions, facility improvements, or special projects focused on the reduction of health disparities.

The disadvantage to public grants is that they generally come with significant degrees of oversight and regulation and a number of stipulations. Also, grant writing requires a great deal of time and energy and any resulting award is uncertain.

STATE AND LOCAL CONTRACTS

Contracts with public entities or other organizations may provide reliable and predictable income for the health center as payment for specific services. Again, public contracts usually come with a great deal of oversight and regulation, and contracts with private organizations, such as other agencies, businesses, unions, city and state governments, or housing authorities, must be constructed carefully to assure that they are specific about services that are covered and those that may be separate from the contract. Contracts cover the ways that disputes are negotiated, and they detail the ways in which services are paid for. Contracts are binding and must be adhered to even if resources or staffing declines, unless both parties renegotiate the terms. See Appendix G for a sample of a contract with a local agency.

Family Planning Contracts

It can be worthwhile to have a contract with the local Family Planning Council if one exists in the area. In Pennsylvania, such a contract awards an annual capitation fee to provider organizations for each patient enrolled in the Family Planning program. The Councils also do the billing to Medical Assistance for contracted family planning providers. Fees are a carve-out fee-for-service arrangement from the managed care Medicaid HMO. The fee-for-service is in addition to the usual capitation for primary care services.

FEE-FOR-SERVICE

The fee-for-service model is a common payment system. It is adjustable in changing financial conditions. However, in setting fees, health centers must find a balance between setting fees that are adequate to cover the cost of services and the need to avoid over-pricing of services, which can significantly reduce the center's financial base. The fee-for-service model requires a billing and collection system and, for many centers, the development of a sliding scale fee schedule for patients who are uninsured or underinsured. The sliding scale is usually based on federal poverty guidelines, and is required to be based on those guidelines for federally funded programs.

THIRD-PARTY REIMBURSEMENT

Third-party reimbursement is another common payment system in health care. There are a number of sources of third-party reimbursement. Medicare, Medical Assistance (Medicaid), insurance companies, HMOs and managed-care organizations, and businesses that contract for certain services are the major third-party payers. The health center should plan according to the mix of payers and rates expected. The mix will vary based on the population served, the services provided, and the sources of payment available. One FQHC in Philadelphia strives to maintain a minimum of 60% Medical Assistance patients, with 30% uninsured and 10% patients insured by Medicare or private insurance. One way this is done is to assist patients to establish their eligibility and apply for Medical Assistance. Medicare now pays a low fee for each visit, but may soon change to cost-based reimbursement rates similar to those for Medical Assistance.

Each payer organization has its own reimbursement policies and fee schedules. It is important to designate one person in the organization who will be responsible for having current knowledge about the reimbursement process of insurers providing third-party reimbursement. Nurse-managed centers will need to obtain a provider number for both Medicare and Medicaid reimbursement. Both of these payers utilize the HCFA1500 form for billing. Depending on the insurance company, provider numbers for these may also be required, so it is important to contact each specific company. For managed-care organizations, providers need to request an application for admission as a new provider.

In some parts of Pennsylvania and other parts of the nation, HMOs and Managed Care Organizations are resistant to contracting with independent nurse practitioners and nurse-managed health centers. Strategic approaches to this issue, spearheaded by the NNCC and nursing leaders, have broken down many of these policies, but they continue to be a barrier in some areas. The approaches include sharing data with the companies that show the least effectiveness and quality of services provided by the health centers. Other approaches include networking with Medical Director and key leadership. It is important for a new health center to explore early on in the planning process the carriers that operate in the area, any limitations that exist to third-party reimbursement for nurse-managed services, and limits on the number of new providers.

The disadvantages of third-party reimbursement are the costly process involved in billing insurers, the sometimes significant delays in payment, and the need to track and follow up on denied payments, Current Procedural Terminology (CPT) codes that may limit reimbursable nursing services, and insurer gatekeepers that may limit the number of new providers (Elsberry & Nelson, 1993). Third-party payment is difficult to obtain for health promotion, disease prevention centers though some centers have received reimbursement for special chronic illness management programs.

Resources for Third-Party Reimbursement:

Abood, S., & Keepnews, D. (2001). *Understanding payment for advanced practice nursing services, volume 1: Medicare reimbursement.* Washington, DC: American Nurses Association.

Buppert, C. (2000). *The primary care provider's guide to compensation and quality: How to get paid and not get sued.* Gaithersburg, MD: Aspen.

Centers for Medicare and Medicaid Services: http://www.cms.hhs.gov/default.asp?

Kaiser Family Foundation website: http://www.kff.org

Managed Care Information Center. (2001). *The National Directory of Managed Care Organizations* (4th ed.). Edited by Lareau, G. B. New York: Health Resources Publications.

Medicare Payment Advisory Commission: http://www.medpac.gov/publications

Part B News: http://www.partbnews.com/pbnweb/index.htm

Summary of Reimbursement Options Under New Medicare Law "Incident To" Provisions: http://www.nurse.org/acnp/medicare/index.shtml

PRIVATE PHILANTHROPIC AND CORPORATE SOURCES

Finding nontraditional sources of funding, such as private philanthropic foundations and corporations, is important because the pillars of public health—health promotion, health education, and disease prevention—are rarely reimbursed by public sources or patients. Yet communities see these services as essential, value-added services. However, because a significant amount of time and management energy needs to be devoted to monitoring and applying for such funding and because the success of such efforts is unpredictable, the organization must consider carefully the pursuit of such funding, and may wish to consider either hiring or contracting for a Development Director. A good Development Director can be extremely worthwhile to an organization.

Before seeking private funding, the organization should complete its strategic plan, as many funders require such a plan before considering a grant, particularly for a new organization or new program. Case statements should also be developed regarding the specific programs or items for which funding will be requested, including a full discussion of the need for the services, details of the services to be provided, outcomes to be achieved, and the methods of evaluation to be used (a sample Case Statement is available on the NNCC website, www.nncc.us). Staff and Board members of the organization should consider collecting quotes regarding the program or services from letters received, phone calls, testimony at public hearings, or comments in the press. These quotes can then be used on the title page of the grant request, as part of a summary paragraph, in the background section of the grant request, or when talking about a specific program. Furthermore, these quotes can be utilized in the annual report or other public relations materials and on the organization's website (Adams, 2002).

In order to identify likely foundation funders, the organization should begin with background research in a directory of foundations (Fazzano, 2002). Starting the search for funders at the local level may be more successful than approaching larger, national foundations. Typically, local foundations tend to fund local organizations. Also, smaller charitable organizations usually have less competition for funds and involve less bureaucracy and oversight (Elsberry & Nelson, 1993). After identifying foundations that share a mission similar to that of the health center, the organization should try to identify people who may know the staff or board members of these foundations. A list of organizations the foundations have funded in the past is usually available and informative. In addition, foundations that currently fund or have previously supported the health center may have leads that will help to diversify the organization's funding. If current donors have contacts with other funders, they may be willing to make some introductions.

Utilizing a personal approach can be helpful in developing a relationship with a potential funder. For instance, inviting a funder to an event is a way to introduce them to the organization's work. Another technique of establishing a relationship is by calling a funder from time to time for advice or technical assistance, if they are receptive to this. It is important to build credibility with grant-makers. Active participation in policy-making activities, advocacy groups, and other organizations can give the health center visibility that will be helpful in the search for support.

Prior to submitting a letter of inquiry, the organization should request the latest application guidelines, an annual report, and other pertinent materials about the funder. The eligibility requirements should be reviewed carefully and the application guidelines should be followed *meticulously*.

There are a number of resources available to assist grant-seekers. The Foundation Center website offers a proposal writing course, foundation directory, and training programs. The Center also offers a book titled *Guide to Grantseeking on the Web*. The Environmental Protection Agency has an on-line grant-writing tutorial that helps the user write more competitive grants. Charity Channel, in partnership with Grant Station, offers a grantsmanship e-newsletter that includes tips, techniques, instructions, and updates in the world of fund raising. To subscribe to this newsletter, go to the website http://www.CharityChannel.com. See Appendix H for a brief list of public and private funding sources.

Resources for Fund Development:

Bureau of Primary Health Care—Funding and Grant Opportunities: http://bphc.hrsa.gov/Grants/Default.htm
Center for Health Services Financing and Managed Care: http://www.hrsa.gov/financeMC
Charity Channel website: http://charitychannel.com/article_892.shtml

Commonwealth Fund: http://www.cmwf.org

Community Health Funding Report: http://www.cdpub
lications.com/pubs/communityhealthfunding

Foundation Center's Proposal Writing Short Course:
http://fdncenter.org/learn/shortcourse/prop1.html

Grant Services Corp. Presentations: http://www.grant
services.com/presentations.htm

Grant Writing Basics: http://www.megrants.org/mpc/
nonprofits/grantwriting.cfm

Hospital Conversion Foundations: http://www.hpolicy.
duke.edu/cyberexchange/conversion/hosconfr.html

Inc. website: http://www.inc.com

Internet-Fundraising website: http://www.internet-fund
raising.com/if2002-08-02.html

LISTSERV@LISTS.FDNCENTER.ORG: Send an e-
mail to this address with the words "Subscribe to RFP
bulletin" to receive weekly e-mails from the Foundation Center about grant opportunities.

Kellogg Foundation: http://www.wkkf.org

Robert Wood Johnson Foundation: http://www.rwjf.org

SmartBiz website: http://www.smartbiz.com

Sportsman, S., & Hawley, L. (2002). *Clinical practice
management strategies for Nurse Practitioners.*

U.S. Chamber of Commerce website: http://www.us
chamber.com

U.S. Small Business Administration website: http://
www.sba.gov

For a frequently updated list of RFPs in health field, see:
http://fdncenter.org/pnd/rfp/health.jhtml

Library of information re fundraising: http://www.map
np.org/library/fndrsng/np_raise/np_raise.htm

Listing of information re fundraising: http://www.lib.
msu.edu/harris23/grants/4fcelec.htm

Prospect research resources (re individual giving): http://
www.lambresearch.com/

Good general resource including announcements of grant
opportunities: http://webnp.nt5.us/

CHAPTER 6

Financial Operations

The operation of a health center requires financial planning and sound financial management. For this reason, it is important for the health center's strategic plan to include a business plan with at least a 2-year projection of revenue, as well as a capital budget and plan. Funding must be identified and secured and financial management processes in place when operations begin.

BUSINESS PLANNING

A Business Plan is a management tool. It helps an organization identify financial and other organizational goals for the year and monitor achievements and setbacks. Before writing a Business Plan, it is important to identify the audience who will be using it, other than the management of the organization. In particular, Business Plans often must be submitted to public and/or private funders as part of proposals for funding or reports on progress made. If an organization's Business Plan will be sent to potential funders, it must be designed to inform them about the organization as well as the goals and objectives for the year. Components of a Business Plan might be:

- Business Description (name, background of the organization, mission of the health center, and special features of the services provided)
- Management Section (organizational structure, roles of key personnel, relevant experience and capabilities of the team, personnel strategies and issues such as recruitment and retention of staff, and service supports such as advisors, boards, and consultants)
- Marketing Section (market research studies completed, market niche, and competitive analyses)
- Financial Section (income statements, balance sheet, cash flow statements, sources and uses of funds, and break-even analysis)

- Critical Risks Section (internal strengths and weaknesses, external threats and opportunities, competitors' strategies, and other possible events that could bring your business to a halt)
- Appendices (purchase orders, contracts, letters of intent, and resumes of management and key personnel)

See Appendix F for a model Business Plan.

FINANCIAL MANAGEMENT

The nurse-managed health center must develop and implement plans to meet the immediate and long-range financial requirements of the health center and manage the organization's fiscal affairs. A long-range financial plan and a capital plan should be part of the strategic plan. As noted above, the organization must seek revenues that are adequate to support the services the health center is committed to provide, including both government and private sources where possible, seeking diversification and balance for stability. Financial procedures should be developed to ensure that the management of health center fiscal affairs is conducted according to sound financial principles and in compliance with all laws related to fiscal accountability and governance. Procedures should be written and used to train financial and management staff.

Budget Development and Monitoring

Creating and following a budget is essential to the survival of the health center. The annual budget should reflect the goals of the health center and should be dynamic so that it can be adjusted to reflect changes in the business and economic environment. The budget should take into consideration funding anticipated during the year, the fixed and incremental costs of operation, and potentially changing costs and conditions. It must also consider the personnel necessary to accomplish long-term and short-term goals and the workloads to be carried by staff members. The development of the annual budget should include a review of the long-range financial plan that is part of the strategic plan. The Board should approve the annual budget before the beginning of each fiscal year. All significant deviations should be explained and the Board should also approve resulting changes.

The annual budget includes revenues, operating expenses including state and federal taxes, and cash flow projections. Revenues are the funds that the organization has and plans to acquire to pay the bills. Operating expenses include rent, insurance, payroll costs, taxes, supplies, building maintenance, interests on loans, and overhead. The budget will help forecast cash needs of the business and control expenditures.

The management and the Board should review fiscal statements no less frequently than quarterly, monthly for FQHCs, to examine the relationship of the budget to actual expenditures and revenues and to examine issues of fiscal policy, budget preparation, and recommendations of the organization's auditors. Reports to the Board should be written and where possible co-presented by a Board member. The Board should also receive reports on practices, trends, and relationships with regard to the agency's part in contractual relationships.

Financial Accountability

Internal audit functions are carried out regularly throughout the year, including cash reports, bank reconciliations, accounts receivable reconciliation, general ledger account analysis, fee and reimbursement collection, and comparison of actual expense to budget. A full audit should be conducted of the governing organization each year by an independent public accountant selected by the Board and should be formally received and accepted by the Board. Any audit recommendations made in the annual audit or by funders should be followed and reported on to the Board.

Financial Procedures

Financial procedures should be designed to provide reasonable assurance regarding the efficiency of center operations, reliability of financial reporting, and compliance with applicable laws and regulations. Procedures regarding internal controls should include but not be limited to:

- Procedures for budget development, monitoring, variance analysis, and audit;
- Procedures requiring an accrual method of accounting and prompt and accurate recording of revenues and expenses;
- Procedures requiring accurate accounts of units of service provided, timely submission, appropriate follow-up on any denial of coverage or payment, and compliance with applicable regulations, which will provide safeguards against over- or under-billing;
- Separation of accounting duties to the extent possible and other methods to prevent and detect fraud or abuse of the controls;
- Procedures for providing reports required by all funding sources;
- Procedures for the review and approval of payroll expenditures, including time and overtime records and written authorization for new hires, terminations, rates of pay, and deductions;
- Authorization levels for all other expenditures;
- Purchasing procedures, including competitive bidding for major purchases;
- Fixed asset procedures and inventory controls; and
- Review and approval of unplanned expenses and for budget adjustments required by variances.

Procedures for FQHCs should also include procedures for the completion of the Uniform Data Set (UDS) report and for unit cost assessment. The use of Medical Group Management software (MGMA) should be considered to assist in required cost analysis. Procedures should indicate that all contracts must be reviewed to assure their compliance with federal requirements and must include language regarding their length and conditions of termination. Contracts for required FQHC services must allow the center to set practice guidelines and review performance.

CHAPTER 7

Policies and Procedures

Policies and procedures guide the work of the health center and promote quality of services, consistency of performance, safety, sound business practices, and communication of standards and expectations throughout the organization. They are essential for providing clear guidelines and rationale for staff practice and behaviors. Health center policies and procedures must be written and should reflect the health center mission, vision, and goals. Involving staff in the development of policies and procedures, whenever practical and appropriate, promotes staff engagement and helps to ensure that they are comprehensive and relevant to staff practice.

The Board should approve the policies of the center. Organizational and Service procedures are developed by health center management to detail how the policies will be implemented. See Appendix I for a sample Table of Contents for a Policy and Procedure Manual.

LOCAL, STATE, AND FEDERAL REGULATIONS

When developing policies and procedures, the health center should be aware of all local, state, federal, and contractual regulations that impact on the operations of the center. State laws govern the scope of practice, prescriptive authority, and collaboration requirements for nurse-managed health centers, while state and federal laws address the care of patients covered by Medical Assistance and Medicare. Governance of Nurse Practitioner practice varies by state and may involve oversight by the State Board of Nursing or joint oversight with the State Board of Medicine. All states require nurse practitioners to hold state licenses as registered nurses and as Certified Registered Nurse Practitioners. Currently, nineteen states require that nurse practitioners have master's degrees and thirty-one states require that nurse practitioners obtain

national certification (Buppert, 1999). The prescriptive authority of nurse practitioners also varies among the states. The Nurse Practitioner's Business Practice and Legal Guide is an invaluable resource for state-specific information (Buppert). Another resource is the State Board of Nursing, an appointed board within each state and territory that regulates the practice of nursing. A list of the State Boards can be found on the National Council of State Boards of Nursing Website. (Go to www.ncsbn.org, then click "Nursing Regulation." Click on "Board of Nursing.") Organizations should stay current on state legislation and be involved in coalitions and task forces that are impacting the rules and regulations that govern nursing practice and health centers.

ORGANIZATIONAL POLICIES AND PROCEDURES

Organizational policies outline the broad management and administrative functions of the health center, delineate the broad responsibilities of staff members, establish such basic requirements as the code of ethics and patient rights, and require the maintenance of quality services. These and personnel policies are approved by the Board. In addition to fiscal procedures that guide the financial operations of the health center, organization procedures include: risk management procedures, personnel procedures, and other administrative procedures including those that guide the management of information and adherence to HIPAA requirements; those that establish processes for patient grievances, reporting of incidents and accidents, reportable illnesses and conditions, and child abuse and neglect; and those that cover other issues, such as cultural competence, management of services to people with hearing or language difficulties, the requirement to establish written collaboration or affiliation agreements, research, inter-departmental referrals, staff travel, public relations and relations with the media, staff development and training, and fundraising.

Risk Management Procedures and Insurance

Health centers should have a risk management plan approved by the Board that assures that required codes are followed, property is maintained well and inspected regularly, safety activities and safety related trainings are carried out, adequate insurances are carried, and Quality Improvement information is used to help reduce organization liability.

Facilities in which health centers are located should meet all required local, state, and licensing codes, as well as Section 504 of the Rehabilitation Act of 1973 and the Americans with Disabilities Act (ADA). Certificates that codes are met and inspections such as those by the Fire Department should be kept on file. Facilities should be inspected regularly based on standards, such as those used by the Joint Commission for Accreditation of Healthcare Organizations, to assure that they are clean, well-maintained, and friendly and welcoming for consumers. Emergency kits and other equipment should be part of the inspections to assure that they are fully stocked with in-date supplies. Also, the requirements of the Occupational Safety & Health Administration (OSHA) need to be followed regarding protection of employees from the possibility of exposure to blood or other potentially infectious materials. Employees must be offered required vaccinations and procedures must be implemented to minimize or eliminate employee exposure to blood-borne and airborne pathogens. OSHA inspectors conduct site visits of health care facilities to ensure that employers are providing a safe work environment.

The risk management plan should outline the use of fire drills, mock codes, and staff training in such areas as infection control and crisis management, as well as field safety for staff who work in the community that will be conducted at least annually. All staff need to be trained in risk management procedures, since they are the first line of defense in identifying problems that could become liabilities for the organization.

Malpractice, Negligence and Insurance Coverage

Adequate insurance coverage is essential for any kind of health services enterprise. There are three types of liability coverage that must be carried: comprehensive general liability insurance for the facility and the organization, officers' and directors' liability insurance, and professional liability, or malpractice, insurance for the health care providers.

Malpractice, according to Buppert (1999), is the "failure of a professional skill that results in injury, loss, or damage," and negligence is "the prevailing legal theory of malpractice liability that includes failure to give necessary care, failure to follow up, and failure to refer when necessary." Familiarity and compliance with practice protocols and guidelines, as well as state law, is one way of preventing lawsuits. Nurse-managed health centers should also be familiar with the regulations of the state regarding the liability of the collaborating physician in the practice and should have knowledge of the guidelines for physicians by law who are required to collaborate with nurse practitioners regarding malpractice lawsuits based on the negligence of the nurse practitioner. See Appendix J for a sample collaborative physician agreement.

According to Henry (1995), nurse-managed health centers should have collaborative practice agreements that define the joint practice roles and responsibilities of nurse practitioners and physicians working together (as cited in Brush & Capezuti, 1997). Because provider roles and responsibilities change over time, these agreements should be reviewed and updated annually to accommodate the shifting roles in the health care system. More information on such agreements can be found at http://www.paco de.com/secure/data/049/chapter18/subchapCtoc.html for Pennsylvania and similar sites for other states. See Appendix K for a sample collaborative practice agreement.

Whether the nurse-managed health center is affiliated with a hospital or university will be one factor in determining the type of malpractice coverage that should be obtained for the nursing professionals employed by the health center. According to Buppert (1999), it is recommended that practitioners have "occurrence" insurance, which covers any incident while the health professional is insured. A "claims made" insurance policy only covers the person when the insurance policy is active, regardless of when the incident occurred. "Tail coverage" can be purchased for a period of time equivalent to the state's statute of limitations for that act of malpractice (Esposito, 2000). Other considerations are the amount of the coverage and the specific acts that are covered by the insurance.

Under the Federally Supported Health Centers Assistance Act, all directly employed staff of Federally Qualified Health Centers funded under section 330 of the Public Health Service Act are eligible to receive medical malpractice insurance through the Federal Tort Claim Act

(FTCA) at no cost to the grantee. The intent of the FTCA was to spare funded health centers costly malpractice premiums. The health center must adhere to quality assurance measures and guidelines, including a credentialing procedure for all health professionals, in order for covered professionals to be protected under this federal government policy. Other health centers will need to purchase private professional liability insurance for their providers. The cost and amount required varies from state to state. Information can be obtained at http://www.hpso.com.

Personnel Policies and Procedures

It is helpful to have someone on the Board or available to the organization who has personnel management expertise. The board, because of their importance to an organization, must always approve personnel policies. The personnel policies should also be published in a manual that is distributed to all employees, with signatures regarding their receipt of the manual and any updates/changes. These policies and their accompanying procedures will help the health center to manage its employees and govern its employment practices in conformity with applicable laws and regulations, including but not limited to the Civil Rights Act of 1964, the Fair Labor Standards Act (as amended by the Equal Pay Act and the Age Discrimination in Employment Act), the Occupational Safety and Health Act, the Americans with Disabilities Act, the National Labor Relations Act, the Family and Medical Leave Act, and the Rehabilitation Act of 1973, as well as applicable state and local laws. Legal counsel should be consulted when personnel policies are developed or revised and when necessary to assure the agency's conformity with legal requirements.

For FQHCs, there are a number of requirements for elements in the personnel manual, including an Equal Employment Opportunity statement and affirmative action plan, conditions of employment, standards of conduct, conflicts of interest, prohibition of sexual harassment, and drug-free workplace notification, among other items.

The organization should determine, through the planning and budgeting process, the appropriate number, qualifications, and credential requirements of the staff needed to carry out day-to-day operations and achieve the goals and objectives of the health center. A written position classification structure with pay ranges should be developed and used for all positions. A benefits package should also be defined and employees kept informed of any changes in it. The organization should carry workers'

compensation insurance, payroll insurance, and health insurance for employees in accordance with state laws and must contribute to FICA for all personnel. It should be determined and stated in policy which staff are eligible for medical insurance, unemployment benefits, tax-deferred accounts, and paid vacation.

Job descriptions that define the experience and qualifications required for the position and specify the duties and responsibilities and outcomes-oriented performance expectations, as well as credentials and other requirements necessary to fulfill the responsibilities of the job, should be maintained for all positions. Job descriptions should clearly state how the employee's work supports the mission of the organization. They are meaningful documents and should be the basis with which to assess each employee's performance. See Appendix L for sample Health Center job descriptions. Care must be taken to assure that positions are properly classified according to Federal Wage and Hour Regulations (Free Clinic Foundation of America, 1998). Procedures for recruitment and hiring should be followed to eliminate, to the degree possible, any discrimination. The procedures of an established organization and such resources as the Internal Revenue Service's website, which provides a helpful tax guide for employers, should be used when developing hiring procedures. Legal counsel should be consulted to assure that all requirements are met. Staffing and hiring should be reviewed regularly to assure that the organization is adhering to the civil rights requirements of many public funders.

Procedures should be followed that assure that all personnel receive a full orientation to the organization, its policies and procedures, and the specifics of their position. Procedures should also specify ongoing training requirements and requirements for annual employee performance review. It may be helpful to develop an affiliation with a health professions training institution to assure that the latest information is available to staff.

In order to hold personnel accountable for their responsibilities, the competence of each employee to fulfill the work responsibilities described in the job description should be assessed through training evaluations and through formal performance reviews conducted at the end of the probation period and annually. Employees perform best when they have the tools they need to do their work, receive regular feedback from their supervisor, and are engaged in their work. Employees are entitled to regular feedback from their supervisor. This should not be limited to the formal annual review but should occur frequently and include concrete examples of how successful the employee is in meeting tasks described in their job description.

FQHCs are required to conduct termination interviews with staff leaving the organization and to use this information and turnover data that is tracked through the quality improvement process to determine if any changes need to be made to improve employee satisfaction and reduce the rate of turnover. Exit interview questions are intended to learn more about the organization as it pertains to employee satisfaction. Questions might include the following: Are you leaving to change your field, obtain a higher salary, obtain a job that the present job does not offer, and what would have to change to prevent you from leaving?

Health Insurance Portability and Accountability Act and Information Management

Administrative policies and procedures must take into consideration the Health Insurance Portability and Accountability Act of 1996 (HIPAA). HIPAA was designed to protect health insurance coverage for workers and their families when they change or lose their jobs, assure the privacy of medical information, and standardize electronic data interchange. The HIPAA Standards for Privacy of Individually Identifiable Health Information, also known as the Privacy Regulations or the Privacy Rules, are a comprehensive set of federal rules aimed at providing confidentiality protection to nearly all medical records and other individually identifiable health information. The Administrative Simplification provisions of HIPAA required that DHHS establish national standards for electronic data interchange and protection of confidentiality and security of health data through setting and enforcing standards. More specifically, HIPAA calls for standardization of electronic patient health, administrative, and financial data. It also requires unique health identifiers for individuals, employers, health plans, and health care providers. Lastly, the act enforces security standards protecting the confidentiality and integrity of individually identifiable health information, past, present, or future.

All health care organizations, health plans, health care clearinghouses, and health care providers must be familiar with HIPAA requirements and comply with them or they face severe civil and criminal penalties ranging from fines to imprisonment. Participation in Medicare and Medicaid also requires compliance with HIPAA requirements. See Appendix M for a sample HIPAA procedure. The HIPAA website is http://www.hrsa.gov/website.htm.

SERVICE PROCEDURES

Each service in the health center, including support services, should have its own set of procedures to guide the staff in the performance of their responsibilities. These procedures should be developed and updated by the director of each program in accordance with good practice and the requirements of the regulators and funding sources of the program. The procedures should be used in the orientation and training of staff and should be formally reviewed by staff and management at least once every 2 years.

Procedures should detail the primary care process, including the requirement to assess patients' health and psychosocial risks and to establish a primary care plan for each patient that integrates primary care services with other services, such as health education, dental, substance abuse, nutrition, and social services. They should include procedures for the provision of all required services; hospital admissions, tracking, and how services are resumed after discharge; the handling of emergencies, patients who are behind in payments, and walk-in patients; and such issues as service eligibility determination, discounts, scheduling, patient grievances, working with handicapped patients, hazardous waste disposal, referrals for services both within the health center and outside, and a drug formulary, where relevant. The procedures required for FQHCs are detailed in the PCER standards. These can be used by all new health centers and should be followed carefully by those wishing to obtain FQHC status.

Clinical Practice Guidelines

Clinical Practice Guidelines are procedures that provide organized methods for analyzing and managing particular diseases or major symptoms. They assure consistent, high quality practice by specifying the scope of nursing practice at the health center, as well as referral mechanisms. It is recommended that a formal mechanism be put in place to update the clinical practice guidelines annually. This mechanism should be spelled out in the policies and procedures.

There are a variety of resources available to aid in the development of such practice protocols. The simplest way is to select an accepted text as the guide for the practice. Some references that could be utilized are *Patient Care Guidelines for Nurse Practitioners* (Hoole, Ouimette, Lohr, Powell, & Pickard, 1999), *Implementing Clinical Practice Guidelines* (Margolis & Credin, 1998), or *Primary Care Medicine* (Goroll, May, & Mulley, 2000). If the health center chooses to use a published manual, the reference needs to be the most current and must have a system for updating the guidelines. Current guidelines are usually available on-line and often HMOs or Managed Care Plans make these available to providers.

Some practices choose to write their own guidelines. The usual format includes the following: definition, subjective, objective, labs, assessment, consultation/referral, plan, diagnosis, treatment, patient education, follow-up, and references. This is time consuming and duplicates much of what is already available.

CHAPTER 8

Continuous Quality/ Performance Improvement

The health center should have a Quality Improvement Plan that is approved by the Board, which details the philosophy, organization, scope, and methodology of the Quality Improvement (QI) program of the organization. This plan and attendant procedures specify a systematic process for monitoring and evaluating the safety, quality, and appropriateness of patient care and identifying and resolving problems. The Quality Improvement Plan should have corresponding sections in the other policies and procedures of the organization. For example, the infection control procedures should state an effective process for monitoring the effectiveness of those procedures, as should the pharmaceutical, laboratory, facility inspection, and other procedures.

The Continuous Quality Improvement process is enhanced by being carried out through a team structure that assures that information gathered regarding the safety and quality of services is shared with and ideas for improvement are sought from as many staff members as possible, contributing to a greater sense of ownership and responsibility.

A structure that is used in many organizations involves quarterly team meetings that include all members of the staff. A representative organization-wide team that may include some Board members and a Management Team then hold meetings where recommended actions are prioritized and approved. Other organizations impart and gather information in regular unit meetings and use a Quality Improvement Committee structure that involves a broad representation from clinical and management staff. Minutes of all QI meetings are kept in a concise action-oriented format. Minutes and supporting materials of representative meetings are available to all staff.

The Quality Improvement process works with four types of information:

- Incidents, accidents and grievances;
- Peer record review and utilization review;
- Stakeholder input; and
- Program evaluation indicators and outcomes data.

This information is compiled and distributed to the teams for analysis and action. Meeting agendas consist of discussion of each type of information, quality improvement projects, and obstacles to quality services.

INCIDENTS, ACCIDENTS, AND GRIEVANCES

Analysis of incidents, accidents, and grievances provides two kinds of information and therefore is reviewed in two different ways. The study of incidents, accidents, and grievances gives the health center information to use for risk management. A pattern of accidents may alert the center to a hazardous condition that should be corrected. A pattern of incidents or grievances could signal that a problem is occurring that could result in lawsuits or in action by a payor. Incidents and grievances also give the center information about the quality of services being provided. A pattern of incidents may indicate to a QI Team that a problem has arisen or that there is a gap in services available to the population served.

PEER RECORD REVIEW AND UTILIZATION REVIEW

Peer record reviews of current and recently closed cases can determine the extent to which health center records and the services they reflect are in compliance with requirements and the quality of the services being provided. It also allows for an independent determination of how well services are being utilized and for the monitoring of resource utilization. Peer record reviews are done on statistically significant numbers of cases by staff who have not been directly involved in or directly supervised the services they are reviewing.

STAKEHOLDER INPUT

Stakeholders fall into three categories: the customer/payors, such as grant-making organizations and third-party payors; the individuals and families served; and the community that the center serves, including area hospitals and specialists with which the health center works. Each team should consider how stakeholders' input will be obtained, including both formal and informal ways that input and guidance may be obtained from the defined community. This input will constitute part of the needs assessment that will assist reviewing the strategic plan.

Individuals served can be surveyed individually or, in some instances, in groups to determine their satisfaction with the services they are receiving. Standardized survey instruments that ensure anonymity should be used where feasible.

PROGRAM EVALUATION INDICATORS AND OUTCOMES DATA

The QI Teams can use two kinds of program evaluation information. The first is the results of inspections of the services by the customer/payors, such as the State, HRSA, or JCAHO. One inspection is the audit carried out by the Certified Public Accountants hired by the Board each year. Problems identified in inspections should be addressed by quality improvement projects that carry very high priority.

The second kind of program information is data gathered regarding each service in the agency. According to Kinsey and Gerrity (1997), data from health promotion, disease prevention, education, outreach, and case-finding activities should all be collected, in addition to primary care and other services provided. Quantitative data are gathered, as well as data selected by each QI Team that can give indication of the outcomes and quality of services provided. The quantitative data indicate the numbers, demographics, and needs of people served and the numbers and types of services provided. This data can be compared with goals set at the beginning of each year. Teams are able to determine whether numeric targets are being met or whether trends are occurring regarding the types of people receiving services. FQHCs are required to gather and review cost and productivity data and software systems are available to help with this process.

In all programs, information should be collected regarding the quality and outcomes of services. Many indicators can be found within clinical procedures and benchmarks are set in the Health Care and/or Strategic Plan. The Bureau of Primary Health Care has also set clinical outcome measures for FQHCs that can be used by any health center. The sample Performance Improvement Plan found in Appendix N is an example. The benchmarks should be reviewed and revised at least annually, using the experience of the center and comparison of results to the experience of others providing similar services to similar populations. Eight nurse-managed health centers in the Philadelphia area are working together on a project that is setting up a common Electronic Medical Record and pooling outcomes data. The results of this project will begin to be available through the NNCC website in September 2004.

OBSTACLES TO QUALITY SERVICE

Time can be taken at QI meetings for discussion of barriers that exist that prevent the health center from providing the highest quality services possible. These discussions might consider outside systems, such as regulators and funders, or internal processes, such as outreach, intake, assessment, and personnel or training issues.

QUALITY IMPROVEMENT PROJECTS

Following discussion of the QI information, what they indicate about the services being provided, and possible causes when they reveal issues of concern, teams determine the Quality Improvement Projects to be undertaken to address issues presented by the information. Quality Improvement projects are designed to:

- Build on strengths,
- Find and replicate good practice,
- Eliminate or reduce identified problems, and
- Implement and monitor the effectiveness of the projects.

Resources for Policies and Procedures:

Campbell, N. J. (1998). *Writing effective policies and procedures: A step-by-step resource for clear commu-*

nication. New York: American Management Association.

Dunphy, L. M. H. (Ed.). (1999). *Management guidelines for adult nurse practitioners*. Philadelphia: F. A. Davis.

Mobley, C. S., & Deutsch, S. (1996). *Medical staff management: Forms, policies, and procedures for health care providers*. New York: Aspen Publishers, Inc.

Page, S. (2002). *Establishing a system of policies and procedures*. Westerville, OH: Process Improvement Publishing.

Resources for Regulations:

ANA Prescriptive Authority Chart: http://nursingworld. org/gova/charts/dea.htm

Resources for Financial Procedures:

McMillan, E. (1999). *Model accounting and financial policies & procedures handbook for not-for-profit organizations*. Washington, DC: American Society of Association Executives.

Resources for Risk Management Procedures and Insurance:

Occupational Safety & Health Administration website: http://www.osha.gov

Aiken, T., O'Donnell, J., & Applebaum, S. (2001). *Nursing malpractice* (2nd ed.). Ed. by Iyer, P. Tuscon, Arizona: Lawyers and Judges Publishing Company.

American Association of Legal Nurse Consultants website: http://www.aalnc.org

American Association of Nurse Attorneys website: http://www.taana.org

Medi-Smart's Nursing Law and Ethics: http://medi-smart.com/law.htm

Nurses Services Organization website: http://www.nso.com

Resources for Personnel Policies and Procedures:

Bernstein, L. (1999). *Creating your employee handbook: A do-it-yourself kit for nonprofits*. Management Center.

Guide for Small Businesses and Other ADA Information: http://www.sba.gov/ada/

Internal Revenue Service—Small Business/Self-Employed: http://www.irs.gov/businesses/small/index. html

States or Commonwealth Workers' Compensation Related Home Pages: http://www.sba.gov/hotlist/work erscompensation.html

Resources for HIPAA:

Administrative Simplification website: http://aspe.os. dhhs.gov/admnsimp

Centers for Medicare and Medicaid Services website: http://www.cms.hhs.gov/hipaa

CMS HIPAA Readiness Checklist: http://www.hipaa.org

Health Information Management newsletter: http:// www.hcpro.com/health-information-management/

Health Privacy Forum: http://www.healthprivacy.org

Health Resources and Services Administration: http:// www.hrsa.gov/website.htm

Phoenix Health System newsletters: http://www.hipa advisory.com

U.S. Department of Health & Human Services website: http://www.hhs.gov/ocr/hipaa

WEDI-SNIP Privacy Policies: http://snip.wedi.org/ public/articles/index.cfm?Cat=17

Resources for Clinical Practice Guidelines:

Abraham, I., Bottrell, M. M., Fulmer, T., & Mezey, M. M. (Eds.). *Geriatric nursing protocols for best practice*. New York: Springer Publishing Company.

American Academy of Nurse Practitioners website: http:// www.aanp.org/default.asp

AHRQ Clinical Practice Guidelines Online: http:// www.ahrq.gov/clinic/cpgonline.htm

Cohen, M. M., & Lanigan, A. (2000). *Nurse practitioner protocols* (3rd ed.). Tallahassee, FL: Sunbelt Medical Publishers.

Goroll, May, Mulley. (2000). *Primary care medicine*. Philadelphia: Lippincott, Williams & Wilkins.

Hoole, Ouimette, Lohr. (1999). *Patient care guidelines for nurse practitioners*. Philadelphia: Lippencott, Williams & Wilkins.

Margolis & Credin. (1998). *Implementing clinical practice guidelines*. Jossey-Bass Inc., Publishers.

Paul, S. (1997). Developing practice protocols for advanced practice nursing. AACN Clinical Issues. *Planning, implementing, and evaluating critical pathways: A guide for health care survival into the 21st century*. In P. C. Dykes & K. Wheeler (Eds.). New York: Springer.

The Process Protocol Workbook for NPs: http://www.npcentral.net/protocol

Star, W. L., Lommel, L. L., & Shannon, M. T. (1995). *Women's primary health care: Protocols for practice.*

W. L. Star (Ed.). Silver Spring, MD: American Nurses Publishing.

State Boards of Nursing: http://www.nursingworld.org/ojin/topic15/bons.htm

CHAPTER 9

Information Systems

Health centers should have data collection systems in place so they are able to demonstrate their impact on clients served, indicate clinical outcomes, and allow participation in research (Barger, 1995). Data collection, particularly on patient outcomes that equate to cost savings to payors, are very valuable in assisting in regulation changes in favor of independent nurse-managed practices. For example, the NNCC has used cost and utilization data to make the case that nurse-managed centers are cost-effective. This data has resulted in policy changes that have lead both Medicaid and private managed care to contract with independent nursing centers.

It is important at the outset to determine what data points need to be collected and what system will be used. Additional questions to consider are what variables to enter, how much should be entered, who enters the data, who will analyze the data, what data funders expect, and what system capacity and equipment are necessary. In addition to tracking client data, the system should also track financial information related to fee collection and third-party reimbursement.

Elements of a practice that a health center's information systems must include are:

- Billing,
- Capitation management,
- General ledger,
- Registration/ enrollment,
- Scheduling,
- Patient tracking,
- Referral tracking,
- Medical records,
- Pharmacy,
- Word processing,
- E-mail,
- Internet access, and
- Spreadsheets.

There are a variety of data collection systems available. If a computer is not available, hand tabulation is an option, but a computerized tracking system has many benefits in terms of aggregating and reporting data.

Microsoft's Access application is the simplest form of standardized data collection. It is a relational database in that a table can be created for each type of information to be tracked. An Access database can collect patient demographics, encounter and service related information, patient satisfaction data, and outcome data such as that collected in the Temple Health Connection 12-Item Health Status Questionnaire. The Microsoft website contains articles and other support features to assist users in learning how to navigate Access. However, Access has some drawbacks such as the inability to perform practice management, lack of nursing intervention documentation, and inability to track or assess clinical outcomes (King, 2002).

To collect comprehensive data and clinical outcomes, Electronic Practice Management (EPM) and Electronic Medical Records (EMR) systems should be considered. In addition to these systems, described below, a report-generation program is needed to produce custom reports and to transfer data from the respective databases into a software program capable of performing statistical operations. This program is extremely important and helpful to the centers in preparing reports for funders.

SPECIALIZED MEDICAL SOFTWARE PACKAGES

An *Electronic Practice Management (EPM) software package* consists of a number of interrelated computer programs that allow the user to schedule patient appointments, send instant messages to the providers, collect and enter patients' demographic and health payer information, enter clinical diagnoses and treatments performed during the visit, generate a paper or electronic bill to send to the payer, enter payments received, and track accounts receivable. Most health care providers today use an EPM because it makes office management functions much more efficient.

An **_Electronic Medical Record (EMR) software package_** consists of a number of interrelated computer programs that enable the health care provider to enter information about their patient's medical history. The EMR, just like the paper chart, contains information about patients' past and current medical problems and their treatments. At each visit, the provider enters health information such as pulse and respiration rates, blood pressure, height, weight, temperature, heart or lung sounds, results of diagnostic tests, etc. Many of the programs also include a feature that reminds the provider to do certain things for the patient, such as recommend that a woman have a mammogram, advise a man to have a PSA test or administer an immunization. Once data are entered, the provider merely needs to type in the patient name to view all the clinical information about the patient—the same kind of information that would be kept in a paper chart.

An EMR has many significant advantages:

- Information is much better organized and more readily accessible than that in a paper chart. For example, if a provider wants to see what kind of heart medication her patient has taken over the course of the past 3 years, the EMR will display a list of both the current and past medications and their dosages.
- Data to assess implementation of the new guidelines and patient outcomes can be extracted from the EMR database to evaluate the impact of a given change in clinical practice on patient health. For example, at the designated date or time frame, an Autochart can prompt clinicians to query a woman aged 50 or older about the date of her last mammogram, and then provide the data entry field in which those data are entered. Similar reminder systems and decision trees for any number of clinical entities can be incorporated, as appropriate, into patient records.
- Once the Electronic Medical Record is implemented, it can also be used as a tool to facilitate dissemination of research findings and to incorporate new practice guidelines based on those findings and agreed upon by the research infrastructure network.

While there are many advantages of using EMR and EPM software systems, there are also some disadvantages.

- These systems can be very expensive, both in initial and ongoing costs. Hardware and licenses for software must be purchased and usually outside consultation is needed to implement new systems. Maintenance and purchasing of up-to-date hardware and changes in software are significant ongoing costs, as are ongoing training and training of new staff.
- Systems can become inoperable, "go down," due to software glitches, temporary suspension of Internet service, or servers that "go down." In any of these situations, clinicians and front desk staff lose their access to the application and to client data, thereby making it extremely difficult to function. Some paper records may need to be maintained so that functioning can continue under these circumstances. Also daily back-ups of the database must be performed. While server and Internet access problems can be expected on occasion, software problems can be minimized by insuring adequate training for staff and selecting a vendor with an excellent reputation for customer service and support.

To select the appropriate EMR and/or EPM systems, the health center first must decide why the product is needed. The main functions of an EPM system are front office interface (e.g., scheduling patients, scheduling providers, and intra-office communication), electronic record, and billing software. Electronic medical records are beneficial in that they improve standardization of documentation, rapid access to specific lab results or other patient reports, and clinical decision support such as reference information regarding treatment guidelines. On the other hand, there are some barriers to EMR implementation. The health center will need a back-up plan for when the system goes down and will need to convince staff members to accept the change involved in implementation. Staff may not be computer literate and may not desire to learn these skills.

In order to be considered for purchase, an EMR software product has to meet a number of criteria:

- The data entry screens must be intuitive, user friendly, and easily navigated to encourage data entry at the point of care. They also must be structured in a manner that minimizes the possibility of data entry errors by providing drop-down lists and check boxes that eliminate or minimize the need for keystroke effort.

- Software should have already developed clinical data-entry templates included for the majority of common pediatric and adult examinations and clinical conditions. Behavioral health templates, while not essential, are desirable.
- The software product must be HIPAA compliant to the extent possible at the time of purchase and has to assure HIPAA compliance as the regulations continue to be refined.
- There must be a mechanism for restricting from view by center staff members certain client data, e.g., data regarding a patient's HIV status.
- The company must be fiscally sound with continual growth in profit and a substantial ongoing investment in product research and development, thereby increasing the likelihood that it would continue to be in business and able to support the software system.
- Data entered in the electronic medical record software must be capable of being exported in a file format that could be read by statistical software such as SPSS or SAS.
- Data entry templates and data fields in the EMR must be capable of being modified by the database administrator to be consistent with variable definitions and variable levels specified by clinical research protocols.
- The cost of buying into the system and the annual maintenance and support costs need to be affordable for low-budget, non-profit nursing centers.
- The software company must have a reputation for excellent customer support and utilize a deployment system that requires minimal maintenance.

The health center will need to establish guidelines to detail medical record maintenance, access to records, consent requirements for release of information and exceptions to those consent requirements, as well as procedures to ensure confidentiality of patients' medical records that comply with the provisions of the Health Insurance Portability and Accountability Act of 1996 (HIPAA). Procedures should also indicate security measures, back-up procedures and requirements that back-ups be stored off-site, as well as a disaster plan in the case of destruction of the facility or system failure.

Resources:

Androwich, I. M., Bickford, C. J., Button, P. S., Hunter, K. M., Murphy, J., et al. (2002). *Clinical information systems: A framework for reaching the vision.* Chicago: American Nurses Association.

EMR vs. paper record comparison: An electronic medical record should still be a medical record. Retrieved on December 27, 2002, from http://www.e-meds.com

Electronic Medical Record Comparisons: http://www.elmr-electronic-medical-records-emr.com

http://www.himss.org/ASP/index.asp

Start Using Microsoft Access: http://www.microsoft.com/office/previous/xp/columns/column06.asp

Mohr, D. N. (2002). Electronic medical records: A guide for clinicians and administrators. *MayoClinic Proceedings, 77*(7), 736.

Safran, C. (2001). Electronic Medical Records: A decade of experience. *Journal of the American Medical Association, 285*(13), 1766.

APPENDICES

A Start-Up Tool Kit

APPENDIX A

Governing Board Bylaws

_____ HEALTH CENTER, INCORPORATED
BYLAWS

ARTICLE I

Principal Office

The principal office of the Corporation shall be at _____, or such other location within the State of _____ as the Board of Directors may determine from time to time.

ARTICLE 2

Purposes

The purposes of the Corporation are to own, operate and maintain a health center for the study, diagnosis, and treatment of human ailments and injuries; to promote medical, surgical, and scientific research and learning; and such other purposes as may be pursued in accordance with the Certificate of Incorporation, as in effect from time-to-time. These purposes for which the Corporation is organized are exclusively charitable, scientific, literary, and educational within the meaning of section 501(c)(3) of the Internal Revenue Code of 1986 or the corresponding provision of any future United States Internal Revenue law.

Notwithstanding any other provision of these articles, this organization shall not carry on any activities not permitted to be carried on by an organization exempt from Federal income tax under section 501(c)(3) of the Internal Revenue Code of 1986 or the corresponding provision of any future United States Internal Revenue law.

ARTICLE 3

Directors

1. _Powers._ The activities, property, and affairs of the Corporation shall be managed by the Board of Directors. It may adopt such rules and regulations as may be required by regulatory authorities.
2. _Elections of Directors._ The initial Board of Directors shall be elected by the incorporator(s). Thereafter, directorships vacant or to be vacant at an Annual Meeting shall be filled by the election of the required number of directors from the candidates nominated in accordance with Paragraph 5 of this Article. Upon demand of any two directors in person, elections shall be conducted by written ballot.
3. _Number and Term of Office._ The Board of Directors shall consist of eleven persons. The number of directorships shall be determined at each Annual Meeting of the Board and from time to time by the Board of Directors. The terms of the directors shall be so fixed that the terms of one-third of such directors shall expire at each Annual Meeting of the Corporation. Approximately one-third of the directors shall be elected each year for a three-year term. No director may serve more than two consecutive terms or six consecutive years.
4. _Composition of the Board._ At least fifty-one percent of the directors must be individuals who utilize the services of the health center as their medical or dental home and they will be known as users of the corporation. The remaining members of the

board, known as non-users, shall complement the user members of the board in terms of technical expertise in areas such as finance, health care delivery, business, law, education, community relations, religion, and investments. Such technical expertise is appropriate to provide oversight to center operations and activities. No more than one half of the non-user members of the Board may earn more than 10 percent of their income from the health field.

5. *Nomination and Election of Directors.* Not less than sixty (60) days prior to each Annual Meeting, the Board of Directors shall elect a Nominating Committee of three (3) directors, who shall determine the number of directorships for the following year. The Nominating Committee, acting by unanimous vote, shall nominate a number of nominees for director equal to the number of directorships that are vacant or will become vacant at the Annual Meeting. In making such nominations, the Nominating Committee shall take into account the requirements concerning the composition of the Board set forth in Paragraph 4 of this Article.

Not less than thirty (30) days before each Annual Meeting, the Nominating Committee shall submit to the Secretary its nominations for directors, and the Secretary shall immediately inform the Board of Directors of these nominations. Not less than fourteen (14) days before the Annual Meeting, any five (5) directors, including at least one consumer/user member, may submit to the Secretary the names of one or more additional nominees ("Alternative Nominees") for director, each of whom shall be designated by them as being alternatives to one of the Nominating Committee Nominees. At the Annual Meeting, the voting procedure followed shall be such that a separate vote is taken for each directorship to be filled, each Nominating Committee Nominee being matched with his/her respective Alternative Nominee(s). Each directorship shall be filled by majority vote of the directors voting (a quorum must be present), except that no nominee may be elected if the effect of such election would be to cause the composition of the Board to be in violation of the requirements contained in Paragraph 4 of this Article.

6. *Expiration of Terms.* Notwithstanding any other provision contained in these Bylaws, the term of office any director shall not expire until his successor has been duly elected and has agreed to serve.

7. *Vacancies.* When any directorship becomes vacant during the period between Annual Meetings of the Corporation, the directors may elect a new director to fill such vacancy until the next Annual Meeting. At such Annual Meeting, such directorship shall be filled as provided in Paragraph 4 and 5 of this Article and for such term as may be appropriate. Nominations to fill such vacancies shall be made by the Nominations Committee, with additional nominations being permitted from the floor.

8. *Director Compensation.* No member of the Board of Directors shall be compensated for their service on the board, although they may be reimbursed for reasonable and necessary expenses incurred for the benefit of the Corporation. Reimbursement shall require the submission of expense vouchers and receipts per corporate travel policies.

9. *Nepotism.* No employee, or relative of an employee by blood or marriage, may serve as a member of the Board of Directors. Relative is defined as mother, father, sister, brother, aunt, uncle, grandmother, grandfather, and first cousin.

ARTICLE 4

Meetings

1. *Regular Meetings.* The Board of Directors shall hold regular monthly meetings pursuant to a resolution of the Board establishing the meeting schedule. If the Board fails to establish such a schedule providing otherwise, it shall hold regular monthly meetings on the fourth _____ of each month. Said meetings shall be held pursuant to written notice given to each director not less than five (5) days before the time set for the meeting, such written notification to include the agenda.

2. *Special Meetings.* Special meetings may be called by the President or by any three directors contacting the President. Special meetings shall be held within or outside of the State of _____.

3. *Telephonic Communication.* Members of the Board of Directors may participate in any meeting of the board by means of conference telephone or similar communications equipment that enables all participants in the meeting to hear each other at the same time. Such participation shall constitute presence in person at the meeting.

4. *Quorum and Voting.* A majority of the directors seated shall constitute a quorum for the transaction of business at any directors' meeting, whether annual, regular, or special. If a quorum is present, the act of a majority of directors voting shall be an act of the Board of Directors, except as otherwise expressly provided in these bylaws.

5. *Notice.* Notice shall be given in writing to each director of each annual, regular, or special meeting of the directors. Such notice shall be delivered by hand, by mail, or by facsimile at least five (5) days before an annual or regular meeting and at least one (1) day before a special meeting. The notice shall state the date, time, place, and purpose of the meeting.

6. *Waiver of Notice.* A written waiver signed by a director, or attendance by a director at any annual, regular, or special meeting, shall be deemed equivalent to appropriate notice and shall be deemed consent to the holding of the meeting.

7. *Attendance.* Any director who fails to be present at three regular meetings of the Board in succession or five (5) for the year, regardless of the reason for the absence, may be removed as a director by the affirmative vote of a majority of the other members of the Board. Any director may also be removed for cause by a two-thirds (2/3) vote of the members entitled to vote.

8. *Conflicts of Interest.* The corporation shall avoid the active participation of any director in a manner that poses a conflict of interest with respect to that director. A conflict of interest shall be considered to arise when any matter under consideration by the Board of Directors involves the potential for a significant or material benefit; or a compensation arrangement exists to a director or any member of his or her immediate family to any business, financial, or professional organization of which the director or any member of his or her immediate family is an officer, director, member, owner, or employee. Whenever any matter comes before the Board of Directors which any director recognizes may give rise to a conflict of interest, the Board of Directors shall not approve any action or transaction bearing upon the conflict unless the following procedures are observed:

a) The affected director or other director(s) shall make known the conflict, and after answering to any questions posed by the other directors, the affected director shall withdraw from the meeting for as long as the matter remains under consideration. Should the matter be brought to a vote of the directors, the affected director shall neither be present nor cast a vote.

b) If the withdrawal of the affected director results in the absence of a quorum, no action shall be taken on the matter until a quorum of disinterested directors is present.

c) The Board of Directors shall not go forward with a transaction or arrangement, in which an affected director acknowledges that a conflict of interest exists, or other directors determine that a conflict of interest exists.

ARTICLE 5

Officers

1. *Officers.* The officers of the Corporation shall be a President, a Vice-President, a Treasurer, a Secretary, an Executive Director, and such other officers as the Board of Directors may from time to time elect. The duties of the officers of the Corporation shall be as provided in this Article, except as modified from time to time by the Board.

2. *Nomination and Election.* The Nominations Committee shall present nominations for the offices of President, Vice-President, Secretary, and Treasurer at each Annual Meeting and at other times when vacancies occur in the offices. Additional nominations may be made from the floor. The President, Vice-President, Secretary, and Treasurer shall be members of the Board and shall be elected to serve for a term of one year and until their successors are duly elected and have agreed to serve.

3. *President.* The President shall preside at meetings of the Board, shall have general responsibility for dealing with questions of policy related to the Corporation's affairs, and shall be responsible for calling meetings of the Board and for assuring adequate communication between the operating staff of the Corporation and the Board on matters of policy.

4. *Vice-President.* The Vice-President shall perform such duties as may from time to time be assigned to him/her by the Board of Directors or designated to him/her by the President. In case of the death, disability, or absence of the President, he/she shall

fulfill all the duties and be vested with all powers and responsibilities of the President.

5. *Secretary.* The Secretary shall keep a book of minutes of all meetings of the Board, shall issue all notices required by Law or requested from time to time by the Board of Directors or by the President, and shall perform such other duties as are incident to the office of Secretary. He/She shall have custody of the seal of this Corporation and all books, records, and papers of this Corporation, except such as shall be in the charge of the Treasurer, Clinical Director, or some other person authorized to have custody and possession thereof by a resolution of the Board of Directors.

6. *Treasurer.* The Treasurer serves as the principal financial advisor to the Board of Directors in planning, directing, and appraising the effectiveness of _____ Health Center's fiscal operations. The Treasurer shall ensure full and accurate accountability and control of the receipts and disbursements of _____ Health Center's assets. The Treasurer shall perform such other duties as may be assigned by the Board of Directors or are incidental to the office.

7. *Executive Director.* The Executive Director shall be appointed or dismissed by the Board of Directors, shall be an ex-officio member of the Board of Directors, and as the Chief Executive Officer of the Corporation shall direct all operations of the Corporation; shall supervise all personnel; and shall have control and management of its business and affairs, all subject to the direction of the Board of Directors. The Board shall evaluate the performance of the Executive Director annually, against a set of written, agreed-upon goals and objectives.

8. *Appointment of Staff.* The Medical and Dental staff of the Corporation shall be appointed at each Annual Meeting by vote of the Board.

ARTICLE 6

Committees

1. *Committees.* Standing committees of the corporation shall include an Executive Committee, a Nominations Committee, a Finance Committee, an Operations Committee, a Bylaws Committee, and a Continuous Quality Improvement Committee. The President, subject to the approval of the Board of Directors, shall appoint members to committees for a term of one year and until their successors have been elected and have agreed to serve. At each Annual Meeting of the Board of Directors, members may appoint other special committees as circumstances may require.

2. *Service on Committee.* The President, subject to the approval of the Board of Directors, shall appoint the chairperson and members of all committees, except as otherwise provided by these Bylaws. Every standing committee and special committee shall include at least one Board member. The terms of office of committee chairpersons and members shall be for one year or until the end of the Annual Meeting following their appointment. No person shall serve more than three successive years as committee chairperson, but there shall be no limitation on the length of time individuals may serve as members of a committee. The President and the Executive Director shall be ex-officio members of all committees except as otherwise provided in these Bylaws.

3. *Executive Committee.* The Board of Directors shall elect an Executive Committee. The members thereof shall be the President, who shall serve as chairman of the Committee, Vice-President, Secretary, Treasurer, and one additional director, who must be a consumer member director. Such one additional member shall be elected to the Executive Committee at each Annual Meeting following the election of directors and shall serve for a meeting; the Nominations Committee shall present nominations for the positions on the Executive Committee to be filled. The Executive Committee shall have power and authority to take actions on behalf of the Board of Directors for emergencies that occur between meetings of the Board. It is intended that the Executive Committee not be utilized to conduct the business of the Board. All actions taken by the Executive Committee shall be reported at the next meeting of the Board and shall be binding on the Board only when approved by formal vote of the Board.

4. *Nominations Committee.* The membership of the Nominations Committee shall consist of three (3) board members appointed by the President. The Nominations Committee shall present nominations for vacancies on the board and for the offices of President, Vice-President, Secretary, and Treasurer at each Annual Meeting and at other times when vacancies occur in the offices. The Nominations Committee will assure that new Board members

receive an orientation to the _____ Health Center and to the role and responsibilities of membership on the Board of Directors.

5. *Finance Committee.*

   a. *Membership*—The membership of the Finance Committee shall consist of the Treasurer and three (3) board members appointed by the President of the Board of Directors.

   b. *Functions*—The Finance Committee shall be responsible to the Board of Directors for the fiscal affairs of the Corporation. Such responsibilities include:

      1) Review, monitor, and approve program budget and recommend changes;

      2) Review and recommend policies regarding financial management activities;

      3) Review and approve all purchases over $5000;

      4) Review and report to the Board on all internal and external audits;

      5) Report to the Board of Directors on _____ Health Center's financial activities; and

      6) Perform other functions as requested of the Committees by the President of the Board of Directors.

   c. *Meetings*—The Finance Committee shall meet at least once each month for the purpose of reviewing monthly financial statements.

   d. *Quorum*—Three (3) members of the Finance Committee shall constitute a quorum.

6. *Operations Committee.* The Operations Committee shall have oversight responsibilities for the development of personnel policies, job qualifications, rates of pay, vacation, and employee benefits, as well as the Strategic Plan and decisions about grant applications and new services. The Operations Committee shall make recommendations concerning the general layout for the physical plant in accordance with the functional needs of the Corporation and shall have general supervision of the upkeep and maintenance of the Corporation's buildings and grounds. This Committee shall have the responsibility for reviewing contracts entered into by the Corporation. Members of the Committee shall prepare for negotiations by becoming familiar with existing contracts at _____ Health Center and current contracts at similar facilities, and developing a knowledge of proper labor management

principles and practices.

7. *Bylaws Committee.* The Bylaws Committee shall make recommendations to the Board of Directors for changes and revisions to the Bylaws and shall meet with a frequency dictated by need or otherwise determined by the Board of Directors.

8. *Continuous Quality Improvement Committee (CQI).* The Continuous Quality Improvement Committee shall develop a system designed to maintain the quality of health care rendered, including a periodic audit of patient records conducted with sufficient frequency to adequately monitor the continuing quality of such care. The CQI Committee will review, approve, and revise as necessary a continuous quality improvement and quality management program commensurate with AMA, ADA, OSHA, and all local, state, and federal regulations. The CQI Committee will also periodically conduct a review of the Board's own performance. The CQI Committee shall meet at least quarterly, or four (4) times per year.

ARTICLE 7

Dissolution

Upon the dissolution of the corporation, assets shall be distributed for one or more exempt purposes within the meaning of section 501(c)(3) of the Internal Revenue Code of 1986, or corresponding section of any future federal tax code, or shall be distributed to the federal government, or to a state or local government, for a public purpose. Any such assets not so disposed of, shall be disposed of by the Court of Common Pleas of the county in which the principal office of the corporation is then located, exclusively for such purposes or to such organization or organizations, as said Court shall determine, which are organized and operated exclusively for such purposes.

ARTICLE 8

Amendments

The Directors may, by a two-thirds vote of those present in person at any duly called meeting at which a quorum is represented, alter, amend, or repeal these Bylaws or any portion thereof, except that Paragraphs 4 and 5 of Article 3 may be altered, amended, or repealed only by the affirmative vote of four-fifths of the directors present.

Written notice as to the substance and effect of any proposed amendment to the Bylaws shall be given or mailed to each director not less than thirty (30) days prior to the meeting of the Board at which such proposed amendment is submitted to a vote.

ADOPTED BY THE BOARD OF DIRECTORS ON

_____.

_____   _____

President   Date
Board of Directors

APPENDIX B

Sample Mission Statement

The Family Practice & Counseling Network

The Health Centers exist to provide quality, comprehensive health services to all the people they serve with special attention to vulnerable people and residents of public housing communities.

The following beliefs guide the work of the Health Centers Network:

- Quality health care is a right, not a privilege.
- Health Centers work best when they are partnerships between consumers and staff.
- Health education is vital to empower individuals to make choices about their health.
- The confidentiality of every consumer's contact with the Centers is a crucial component of providing quality care, and is the responsibility of all center staff.

- No one will be turned away because of an inability to pay.
- Health care must be delivered in a competent, sensitive, and compassionate manner by caring for the whole person—body, mind, and spirit.
- The Health Center Network environment should nurture the staff and encourage their best performance by fostering creativity, commitment, and engagement.
- The Health Center Network will maintain a fiscally sound operation.
- The Health Centers will strive to be exemplary models of nurse-managed community based health care.

The Health Centers are programs of Resources for Human Development, Inc.

Appendix C

Sample Strategic Planning Policy

Purpose: This policy outlines the strategic planning process that the Family Practice and Counseling Network conducts in order to:

- Clarify the mission, values and mandates of the Network;
- Assess the strengths, weaknesses, opportunities, and threats of the organization;
- Establish goals and objectives, which flow from the mission and the Network's mandated responsibilities;
- Assess financial and human resources needs; and
- Identify and formulate strategies to meet identified goals.

Policy: At least every 4 years, the Network will conduct a system-wide, long-term strategic planning process. The Management Team will work with the Advisory Board to develop the strategic plan. The process will begin with a strategic analysis, which will include a needs assessment and, using the information gathered in the needs assessment and the ongoing quality improvement process, an analysis of the Network's strengths, weaknesses, opportunities, and threats. Then a Board and Management retreat will be held where the future directions of the Network, including goals, objectives, strategies, and resource needs, will be developed.

The Advisory Board, as well as the Board of RHD, will review the final Strategic Plan and approve it. The Strategic Plan will be part of the Board Manual distributed to all Advisory Board members and will be given to staff members as well.

Procedures: Needs Assessment

An extensive community needs assessment will be conducted that will include demographic information regarding the areas and populations served and will examine trends in the systems in which the Network functions and changes that have taken place or are projected. The needs assessment will include the development of demographic profiles of the community served and the actual population of persons being served.

The needs assessment will also include surveys of stakeholders— persons served, staff, RHD board and management members, members of the Network's Advisory Board and advisory committees, volunteers, community representatives, contractor organization, and referral source staff—to determine:

- Their perceptions of changing community conditions, trends, and needs, particularly in areas that the Network may be able to address; and
- Their opinions of the Network's current performance and what the Network could do to improve services.

SWOT Analysis

The Network will conduct an analysis of its Strengths, Weaknesses, Opportunities, and Threats (SWOT), using the information gathered in the Quality Improvement process and the needs assessment.

The Advisory Board and as many staff members as possible will be involved in a series of meetings where the SWOT analysis will be conducted. The information generated will be distilled into an integrated analysis that will identify the strategic issues facing the organization, which will be distributed to all of the people who will participate in the planning retreat that will generate the elements of the final Strategic Plan.

Strategic Plan Structure

The Strategic Plan will briefly discuss the reason and process for the development of the Plan and then will consist of three sections: the History, Mission, Population, and Services of the Network; a Strategic Analysis of the Network's Current Position, including the Strategic Issues determined at the retreat; and the Network's Future Directions, including goals and objectives, strategies for achievement, resource requirements, designation of responsibility, and timeframes. An Executive Summary may be included, as well as detailed appendices, which may include:

- Description of Strategic Planning Process—A description of the process used to develop the plan, who was involved, minutes of the retreat, and any major lessons learned to improve planning the next time around.
- Strategic Analysis Data—The detailed information generated during the needs assessment and the SWOT analysis.

- Budget Plan—The detailed description of the resources and funding needed to achieve the strategic goals.
- Health Care Plan—A description of the service goals and activities to be accomplished over the coming year in the format required by HRSA.
- Business Plan—A description of the operational goals and activities to be accomplished over the coming year in the format required by HRSA.
- Quality Improvement Plan—A description of the detailed process for monitoring and improving the services of the Network.

APPENDIX D

Sample Strategic Plan

TABLE D.1

Goal	Objectives	Strategies	Resources	Responsibility	Timeframe
Expand medical specialty services Implement process for consideration of new services/major ideas	Write procedures re: Catalyst sends idea to PCD. Considered within 2 weeks by management team/ PCC group. Planning group identified for approved ideas. Catalyst gets feedback	Identify planning group		Management Team	2/04
	Train staff on new process				3/04
Implement services currently known to be needed	Have dental services at 11th Street and Falls that are available to Abbottsford and Health Annex	Implement current grant	$$$ Funds Space/equipment Provider partner Knowledge re: billing	Patty (11th St) Donna (Abb) and fiscal rep.	1/04
		Apply for state/HRSA oral health grants	Grant writing assistance, Dental Director 11th St	Patty and Donna	12/05
	Have podiatry services in all sites	Identify planning group		Catalyst(s) and PCND	12/05
		Find and hire or contract with podiatry provider	Space/equipment Fiscal knowledge Provider partner		1—12/03 2—4/04 3—10/04
	Increase capacity to provide nutrition education and resources to the community at each center	Identify planning groups at Health Annex, 11th Street. Explore availability of Resources for Human Development (RHD) nutrition specialist	Nutrition expert Educational materials Community resources/ insurance Referrals from NPs and Behavioral Health (BH)	RNs and outreach workers	6/04

54

TABLE D.1 *(continued)*

Goal	Objectives	Strategies	Resources	Responsibility	Timeframe
Expand and Integrate Behavioral Health Services					
Maximize current staff resources	Meet quotas for billable hours/ decrease rates of no-shows/ cancellations, increase productivity standards (# of visits expected per provider)	Improve efficiency by: Scheduling regular no-shows for 1/2 hour sessions. Scheduling therapists so more hours are booked	Behavioral health directors who serve similar populations, David Dan, Alan S.	Sarah, Lynn, and Carolyn, with Medical Director where needed	
	Improve interface and coordination with Primary Care (PC) providers	Join PC to get case management help from HMOs and identify when patients are ready for BH		BH managers with PC providers	
		Use case managers to follow up on compliance issues and do non-therapy but necessary services, e. g., advocacy, food, housing		BH managers with outreach	
	Streamline paperwork	Revise existing forms		BH managers	
		Develop and use an EMR	EMR system Hardware	BH managers with IT help	
Create BH infrastructure for improved service delivery	Improve interface and coordination with PC providers about cases	Restructure team meetings to better address clinical and administrative needs with PC at each site		Sarah, Lynn, and Carolyn, with Medical Director where needed	12/03
	Assure that all staff are clear on areas of responsibility and accountability for operations, treatment coordination, and crisis management	Create and/or revise policies and procedures (incl. charting, scheduling, treatment coordination, crisis management) to assure clear internal communications			6/04
Expand range and capacity of services	Provide more Mental Health (MH) support services, e.g., groups, community-based programs	Apply to HRSA for funding for this type of activity	Grant-writing assistance	Sarah, Donna	12/05

(continued)

D. Sample Strategic Plan

Goal	Objectives	Strategies	Resources	Responsibility	Timeframe
Expand and integrate outreach/social services					
Increase effectiveness of outreach services	Create and maintain outreach/social work department infrastructure	Identify planning group			12/03
		Identify community programs social worker	$$$ Funds		
	Share resources between Network sites	Create resource guide re: what is available at each health center	Design/printing		9/04
		New Abb-Falls outreach coordinator will have formal mentoring relationship with Fran from 11th St.		Fran, Erin	10/03
		Community resource guide re: government services, community social services—both local to each site and for larger community	Design/printing		9/04
	Expand on role as bridge connecting clinical and BH	Improve communication between NPs, therapists, and outreach workers re: status of individual patients (report at NP meeting or joint meeting w/Behavioral Health, Nurse Practitioner, Social Worker			9/04
		Education/training— initial and ongoing for outreach workers. Also orientation to health centers/nurse management model/philosophy			9/04
	Create pool of community volunteers—individuals and organizations. Match volunteers, staff with strengths and interests	Identify planning group			12/03
Increase visibility and range of outreach/social work services	Increase distribution of pamphlets, brochures, revisions, design, professional looking	Identify planning group to design Network materials and approve those designed by sites to assure that they are professional looking	Stuff—i.e., brochures, cups, T-shirts, refrigerator magnets, health ed materials (Network and site specific)		9/04
	Outreach vehicle separate from patient transportation with Network/Health Center identification		$$$ Funds		9/04
	Add services as ideas arise	Develop process for consideration and implementation of new ideas	$$$ Funds Program space (at sites or in community), storage for stuff, offices for outreach/social work staff		9/04

TABLE D.1 *(continued)*

Goal	Objectives	Strategies	Resources	Responsibility	Timeframe
Improve communication	Improve communication among Advisory Board members	Leave open discussion period on Board meeting agenda		Donna/Manya	10/03
	Improve communication between Advisory Board and management	Solicit agenda items from Board in meeting notices		Donna/Manya	10/03
		Send interim mailing to Advisory Board members that provides current report on key Network issues		Donna/Manya	12/03
	Improve communication between staff and management	Each standing committee will review its schedule and use of meeting time to assure that meetings are meaningful and contribute to communication		All standing meetings	12/03
		E-mail key issues from each senior management meeting to all staff		Donna	9/03
		Hold strongly encouraged all staff meetings/events		Management Team	At least 2/year
		Establish an RHD "Citizen Advocate" type of process		Donna, Wayne, Mary Murphy	12/03
	Improve communication among centers and disciplines	Establish an intranet bulletin board	IT capacity Staff training	Donna, Management Team	???
		Other strategies per staff suggestions in 10/03 all staff meeting		All staff	12/03
Revise and clarify organizational infrastructure	Finalize organizational chart with relationships	Assure that lines of communication are clear		Management Team	12/03
		Info gathering to include all centers and levels			
	Review and revise policies and procedures	Ann D. will draft revised policies and procedures. Donna will review and bring revisions to Senior Management Team with subgroups created for review discussion and finalization. To be decided: Which are all the same? Which are site-specific?		Management Team	6/04
		Training to include cross-training for functions/centers			

(continued)

Goal	Objectives	Strategies	Resources	Responsibility	Timeframe
Expansion of Network **Expansion of physical space in existing sites and/or new sites**	Expand physical space in existing sites as needed	Donna will present recommendations to the Management Team and Advisory Board for discussion and input. Donna and RHD will make final decisions.		Donna, RHD, with input from the Senior Management Team and Advisory Board	10/03
	Continue at current number of sites for 2 years unless there is a reason to consider a new site. Decision process will consider environment and the fiscal soundness of the Network.	Donna will present recommendations to the Management Team and Advisory Board for discussion and input. Donna and RHD will make final decisions.		Donna, RHD, with input from the Senior Management Team and Advisory Board	10/03
Raise additional funds and obtain lobbying and PR assistance	Form a fundraising/lobbying/PR committee	Donna to meet with Sue H. and Phyllis B. to plan first brainstorming session; Donna to meet with key people		Donna, Patty, Peggy	11/03
		Bring idea people/key people in community to an event to brainstorm with us re: projects/hooks, people, methods	Facilitator	Donna, Patty Adv. Bd. members	12/03
	Create and implement a Development Plan	Consider ideas, i.e., capital campaign to add space to a site to expand service, child BH Tangible, engenders passion Goal/project-oriented Opportunity to give personally	Consider hiring a professional part-time	Donna, Patty, Peggy	3/04
Expand and improve the Information Technology capacity of the Network					
Implement an EMR/practice mgmt/billing system integrated across sites/disciplines	Implement MYSIS EMR system	Build templates for Primary Care		Deb	11/03
	Develop IT department for the network	Plan hiring process and hire IT professional	$$$ Funds	Deb, Mary, Peggy	10–11/03
	Systematic enhancement and maintenance of system	Review/develop/monitor IT system		IT professional with Deb, Mary	1/04

TABLE D.1 *(continued)*

Goal	Objectives	Strategies	Resources	Responsibility	Timeframe
Maximize the use of technology to improve communication among sites and disciplines	Network all four sites –e-mail –website with shared files –computer maintenance			IT professional with Deb, Mary, Peggy	6/04
	Explore implementation of EMR across disciplines (BH, podiatry, Certified Nurse Midwife [CNM], etc.)			IT professional with Deb, Mary, Peggy	12/05
Maximize use of technology to communicate with the community	Development, maintain, and monitor website			Kyle, Mary	12/03

APPENDIX E

Sample Health Care Plan

_____—New Access Point Health Plan

Problem/Needs Statement: Low-income minority groups who reside in economically declining _____ neighborhoods unfairly bear the burden of disease and other adverse health conditions and face premature disability, morbidity, and mortality. There are no FQHCs in the target area that has 37% of the population at or below 200% of poverty and where 41. 3% of poor adults estimate their health as fair to poor.

TABLE E.1

Goals/Objectives Healthy People 2010 (HP)	Key Action Steps	Data Source & Evaluation Method	Outcome & Measurement	Person/Area Responsible	Comments
A. Increase access to high-quality health care.					
A.1. Provide all required FQHC services at Hill Creek.	A.1.(a) Immediately initiate primary health and behavioral health services on site.	A.1.(a) Client records document services provided, referrals, follow-ups and case management.	A.1.(a) Regular audits of client records, Managed Care Organizations (MCOs) reports, Community Board feedback, & client satisfaction will document client outcomes and quality performance indicators (Health Pro Software Program).	A.1.(a) Director, Primary Care Clinical Coordinator, Practice Manager, in place medical consultation contract with Community Health Associates (CHA)	A.1.(a) Upgrade computer system to support all FQHC reporting requirements.
	A.1.(b) Improve physical plant to support anticipated high facility use by end of Year 1 and be aesthetically pleasing.	A.1.(b) Physical plant improvements by Year 1 appropriate for high use health care facility.	A.1.(b) Staff and clients report on plant improvements that are attractive to all and maintain safety and security measures.	A.1.(b) Director, Practice Manager & Primary Care Clinical Coordinator & Community Board	A.1.(b) Consult with Community Board, Philadelphia Housing Authority, __U about timelines, material selection, installation and functionality.
	A.1.(c) Provide on-site primary heath care to a minimum of 1,646 clients Year 1 and 1,977 Clients Year 2.	A.1.(c) Review of client records and computerized data.	A.1.(c) On-site provision of primary health care to targeted number of clients through new access point.	A.1.(c) Primary Care Clinical Coordinator, Family Nurse Practitioners, Support Staff	A.1.(c) Client Flow and staff productivity monitored daily, weekly, monthly by Practice Manager with Primary Care Clinical Coord.

Problem/Needs Statement: Low-income residents of targeted public housing complexes suffer from significant health disparities in the areas of mental health, substance abuse problems, dental health etc. Thirty-three percent of Health Center residents rate their health status as poor and many report that they have had one or more episodes of "sadness" during the past year and have sought relief through illicit drug or substance abuse (i.e. alcohol and/or tobacco). Benign neglect of dental health is evident with more than 50% of children and 30.6% of poor adults reporting no dental care due to cost.

TABLE E.2

Goals/Objectives	Key Action Steps	Data Source & Evaluation Method	Outcome & Measurement	Person/Area Responsible	Comments
A. Increase access to high-quality health care.					
A.1. Provide all required FQHC services at ———————— Health Center @ Hill Creek or through linkage with HRSA PHPC site or FQHC site.	A.1.(d) Provide on-site Behavioral Health, Mental Health, Substance Abuse Counseling Services to a minimum of 75 clients per year. A.1.(d).1 Utilize depression screen (primary care providers), counsel & refer to onsite therapist.	A.1.(d) Audit of client records and related data such as referrals/reports from supporting organizations/consultants and supervisors. Review of transportation logs for needed referral made services.	A.1.(d) On-site provision of behavioral health services to a minimum of 75 clients per year with anticipated range of 5 to 8 encounters per client (individual counseling and small group work), 150 clients over two years.	A.1.(d) Behavioral Health Therapist, Primary Care Clinical Coordinator, Practice Manager and Abbottsford Behavioral Health Program Psychologist Supervisor	A.1.(d) Commitment in place for linkage with HRSA-funded PHPC site (——————) for Behavioral Health supervision. A.1.(d).1 Transportation support in place A.1.(d).2 Monthly review of depression screens & client outcomes (referrals, kept appointment).
	A.1.(e) Refer a minimum of 200 clients to City of ———————— Department of Health Center 9 for dental health services yearly.	A.1.(e) Review of client records, Health Center 9 reports, client feedback, and transportation logs.	A.1.(e) 347 or more appointments kept for dental health care provided through formalized linkage with Health Center 9 by Year 2.	A.1.(e) Primary Care Clinical Coordinator, Support Staff, Outreach Public Health Nurse	A.1.(e) Linkage with other funded HRSA site in place. A.1.(e).1 Transportation support in place.
	A.1.(f) Provision of age-appropriate primary health care services according to FQHC standards, HP 2010 and U.S. Preventive Services Task Force Report. Screen for substance abuse, mental health needs & refer.	A.1.(f) Review of client records and MCOs data. Utilize Community Health Indicators provided by PHMC as comparative data.	A.1.(f) 90% or more of enrolled clients will receive primary care services in accordance with the U.S Preventive Task Force Report.	A.1.(f) Primary Care Clinical Coordinator and designees	A.1.(f) Regularly scheduled clinical conferences, continuing education meetings and attendance at Public Housing Conferences to increase staff knowledge/skills.
			A.1.(f).1 Refer clients as needed to community resources.	A.1.(f).1 Social Worker, Behavioral Health Therapist	

Problem/Needs Statement: Thirty-five to fifty percent of uninsured, low income, minority children and adults present for care each month and have no local access to essential diagnostic services, affordable medications, and linkages to indigent drug programs.

TABLE E.3

Goals/Objectives	Key Action Steps	Data Source & Evaluation Method	Outcome & Measurement	Person/Area Responsible	Comments
A. Increase access to high-quality health care					
A.1. Provide all required FQHC services at _____ Health Center @ Hill Creek or through linkage arrangements.	A.1.(g) Provide diagnostic laboratory services for all clients and diagnostic x-ray services through _____ Medical Center, or _____ Health Centers 9 or 10.	A.1.(g) Review of client records and laboratory logs.	A.1.(g) Clients receive required laboratory & diagnostic tests.	A.1.(g) Primary Care Clinical Coordinator	A.1.(g) CLIA Level I laboratory place. Special Waiver in place for Level 3 Lab for Blood Lead Analyzer for lead toxicity.
	A.1.(h) Purchase/Distribute pharmaceuticals through Federal Drug Pricing Program to clients with no prescription coverage.	A.1.(h) Review of client records, monitor usage.	A.1.(h) Eligible clients receive prescribed drugs without charge.	A.1.(h) Primary Care Clinical Coordinator, Social Worker, PHN Case Manager	A.1.(h) Social Worker will enroll users in Emergency Indigent Pharmaceutical programs when eligible.
A.2 Identify outreach sites for marketing new access point. Build upon and extend current relationships through PHA and community linkages.	A.2.(a) Conduct weekly outreach, public service announcement campaigns, community programs in public housing and designated neighborhoods sites to inform of new access point, sliding fee schedules, insurance contracts and services.	A.2.(a) Monthly review of outreach activities and community feedback logs.	A.2.(a) A minimum of 52 outreach programs or presentations and 4 public services announcements (PSAs) will be done in Year 1 and 2. Programs will reach 3,000 or more people. PSAs will reach 350,000 viewers.	A.2.(a) Director, Practice Manager, Primary Care Coordinator, Outreach Public Health Nurse, and others at site and Community Board	A.2.(a) Outreach sites are identified for marketing new access point. Current relationships will be built upon and extended through PHA and community linkages. Public Services Announcements (PSAs) will be produced for University Channel 56.

Problems/Needs Statement: To address the notable health disparities of minority groups, specifically African-American, Hispanic, and Asian populations, by increasing the provision of culturally competent primary health care. Target population includes core area which is 52.4% Black, 15.3% Hispanic, and 13.15% Asian.

TABLE E.4

Goals/Objectives	Key Action Steps	Data Source & Evaluation Method	Outcome & Measurement	Person/Area Responsible	Comments
A. Increase access to high-quality health care.					
A.3. Enroll new users and provide culturally competent care.	A.3.(a) Enroll clients in the _____ Health Center at Hill Creek primary care new access site.	A.3.(a) Review of appointment logs, new appointments kept, no-show rates, and client records.	A.3.(a) Year 2, the number of enrolled clients will exceed 1,977 people of all ages.	A.3.(a) All key personnel	
	A.3.(b) Ensure clients return for recommended follow-up services through case management and tracking system for recalls and no-shows.	A.3.(b) Review client records, appointment calendars, and referral systems.	A.3.(b) 90%+ of clients who do not keep first appointment and those who miss have return appointments. Have one or more contacts to reschedule & address barriers to care.	A.3.(b) Primary Care Clinical Coordinator	A.3.(b) National Nursing Centers Consortium and the *PA Forum for Primary Care* are resources to examine new access point issues.
	A.3.(c) Ensure provision of culturally competent, linguistically appropriate care.	A.3.(c) Review of client, community profiles; examine utilization patterns of translation and interpreter services.	A.3.(c) All staff has one or more Cultural Competency Trainings per year plus on-site clinical conferences.	A.3.(c) Director, Practice Manager, Primary Care Coordinator	A.3.(c) Utilize HRSA Cultural Competence Training Program with other similar organizations & other conferences to build staff skills. A.3.(c).1 In-place translation and interpretation services.

Problems/Needs Statement: Citywide 31% of African-American women had no prenatal care in 2002 and a disproportionate number of _____ women have late entry into prenatal care. The teen pregnancy rate in the catchment area is 83 as compared to 70 citywide. 100% of minority women access prenatal services at the Health Center site (predominately African American) and 90% have no health insurance at the time of the first visit.

TABLE E.5

Goals/Objectives	Key Action Steps	Data Source & Evaluation Method	Outcome & Measurement	Person/Area Responsible	Comments
A. Increase access to high-quality health care.					
A.4. Maximize the number of pregnant women who enroll in prenatal care during the first trimester.	A.4.(a) Outreach to target groups in schools, nutrition sites, public assistance offices, and other settings where childbearing aged women reside or work.	A.4.(a) Outreach logs, site contact feedback forms reviewed monthly.	A.4.(a) 150 or more pregnancy tests provided at new access site annually.	A.4.(a) Primary Care Coordinator, Nurse Practitioners, Nurse Midwives	A.4.(a) In-place Nurse Midwifery Contract with _____ Medical Center for Nurse midwife services.
	A.4.(b) Prenatal & postpartum services provided on site through Prenatal Contract with _____ Women's Health/ _____ Medical Center Women's Health Center	A.4.(b) Healthy Beginnings Plus Records & user charts reviewed monthly.	A.4.(b) 20 or more childbearing women registered for first trimester care during Year 1 and 70% keep all appointments. 38 women or more during Year 2 and 75% keep all appointments. (9 to 11 visits are target)	A.4.(b) Primary Care Coordinator, Nurse Midwives, Prenatal Nurse Practitioners	A.4.(b) In place PA. Site Provider for Healthy Beginning Plus (Medicaid site). Midwifery sessions increase in Year 2.
	A.4(c) Delivery and neonatal services coordinated by staff for enrolled users at _____ MC.	A.4(c) Client delivery records, social work records, _____ MC records reviewed monthly.	A.4(c) 90% of users deliver at term at _____ MC, return for post-partook care, make and keep appointments for their newborns at Hill Creek site.	A.4(c) Primary Care Nurse Coordinator, Nurse Midwives, Prenatal Nurse Practitioners, PHN & SW Case Managers	

Problem/Need Statement: Infant mortality rate of 16.7 per 1,000 live births in the target area with low birth weight rate of 116 as compared to 109 citywide.

TABLE E.6

Goals/Objectives	Key Action Steps	Data Source & Evaluation Method	Outcome & Measurement	Person/Area Responsible	Comments
B. Improve maternal/child health.					
B.1. Improve pregnancy outcomes.	B.1.(a) Identify and enroll low-income first-time childbearing women in nurse home-visit program that supports client through pregnancy and family for first 2 years of infant's life.	B.1. (a) Nurse-Family Partnership Program Record Review: weekly, monthly, quarterly.	B.1.(a) 100% of clients enrolled in prenatal programs in catchments area with 30% enrolled at Hill Creek site & 95% referred for community services.	B.1.(a) Director, Nurse Midwifes, PHN Case Manager	B.1.(a) Nurse Family Partnership Program Collaborative is an enhancement to the new access site. Director administers _____ TANF grant for nurse home-visit collaborative.
	B.1.(b) Clients in program deliver healthy newborns. B.1.(c) Clients referred to essential community resources (WIC, MA).	B.1.(b) Delivery room logs review monthly. B.1.(c) Referrals recorded on record & reviewed.	B.1.(b) 90% of infants born are at term and average weight. B.1.(c) 85% of referrals made are kept.	B.1(b) Director, Nurse Midwives, PHN Case Manager B.1.(c) PHN Case Manager	
B.2. Improve infant and child health	B.2.(a) Newborn and follow-up pediatric appointments made and kept.	B.2.(a) Review records monthly.	B.2.(a) 90% newborn appointments kept with 30% or more enrolled at Hill Creek site.	B.2.(a) Primary Care Nurse Coordinator, Director, Primary Care Coordinator, PHN Case Managers	B.2.(a) Barriers to access to care to other providers documented and interventions developed (i.e., tokens & taxi vouchers).
	B.2.(b) Infants in Nurse Family Partnership Program up-to-date with immunizations & Early Periodic Screening Diagnosis and Testing for children and adolescents age 0 to 21 years.	B.2.(b) Review records quarterly.	B.2.(b) 85% or more of infants in program are immunized on time with age-appropriate EPSDT.	B.2.(b) Primary Care Provider, Nurse Practitioners	B.2.(b) Barriers to on-time immunizations & EPSDT screens documented & analyzed.

Problem/Needs Statement: The target area is fourth highest for child abuse and neglect according to City of _____ Department of Health & Human Services indicators.

TABLE E.7

Goals/Objectives	Key Action Steps	Data Source & Evaluation Method	Outcome & Measurement	Person/Area Responsible	Comments
B. Improve maternal/child health					
B.2. Improve infant and child health	B.2.(c) Focus on healthy child development and provide child abuse, neglect screens during primary care and home-visit services.	B.2.(c) Review of client records and home-visit records.	B.2.(c) 5% or less of clients in Nurse Family Partnership Program are referred to child protective services.	B.2.(c) Primary Care Coordinator, Social Worker, PHN Case Manager	B.2.(c) Tokens for transportation to Hill Creek site will increase site use by clients.
	B.2.(d) Provide on-site childbirth and parenting classes.	B.(d) Review of client logs, evaluation forms, and pregnancy outcomes.	B.2.(d) 50% of enrolled midwifery clients participate in on-site sessions and 70% participate overall in childbirth education.	B.2.(d) Nurse Midwives, PHN case manager and select personnel	B.2.(d) _____ MC provides childbirth education classes. Selection of time & site optional for client.
	B.2.(e) Provide parenting classes on-site and in select community settings and provide individual counseling sessions for clients with time management issues.	B.2.(e) Review of client logs, evaluation forms and other data.	B.2.(e) 20 clients participate yearly in parenting sessions on site. 100 women in Nurse Family Partnership Program receive ongoing parenting support.	B.2.(e) Director, Primary Care Nurse Coordinator, Nurse Midwives, PHN Case Manager	B.2.(e) Monitor Department of Human Services reports regarding child abuse and neglect cases and substitute care placements.

Problem/Needs Statement: Public school health data document that 30–40% of preadolescents/adolescents need ongoing primary health care and required immunizations and display risky behaviors (smoking, illicit drug use, sexual activity, family violence). Majority of 8th grade public school children cannot read or compute at grade level. Public housing heads of households report absence of organized youth activities and further need for self-esteem, positive decision-making programs that guide health behaviors and career goals.

TABLE E.8

Goals/Objectives	Key Action Steps	Data Source & Evaluation Method	Outcome & Measurement	Person/Area Responsible	Comments
C. Improve pre-adolescent & adolescent health.	C.1.(a) Outreach to schools, recreation centers, and family centers in target area to inform of new site and supportive education services to parents & adolescents & available insurance options.	C.1. (a) Review of monthly outreach logs, feedback from school nurses & other community members.	C.1.(a) Outreach to 40 sites or more yearly. 3,000 or more children informed of programs & access sites.	C.1.(a) Director, Outreach PHN, Primary Care Clinical Coordinator, select staff	C.1.(a) In-place school relationships established through prior HRSA support. C.1.(a).1 Uninsured youth enrolled in CHIPLINK for care & Stepping Stones program for insurance.
	C.1.(b) Provide educational programs for target youth groups.	C.1.(b) Self-esteem, positive decision-making, health career, tutoring programs in place on-site or at community site.	C.1.(b) 300 or more youth involved in self-esteem, tutoring, health career programs.	C.1.(b) Outreach PHN, Social Worker, PHN Case Manager	C.1.(b) Bridging the Gap Health Professional program in place for Hill Creek children/youth in summer session. LSU student tutoring at Hill Creek/Fall & Spring, William Penn Foundation Youth Opportunities Initiative, Reach for the Stars in place.
	C.1.(c) Design/provide primary care access site hours for youth for well checkups, immunizations, special concerns.	C.1.(c) Primary care hours for youth for immunizations, posted at site, in schools.	C.1.(c) 200 or more pre-adolescent/adolescent youth receive one or more primary care service on-site per U.S. Preventive Task Force.	C.1.(c) Primary Care Clinical Coordinator	C.1.(c) Utilization patterns examined & strategies to further engage underserved youth in place.

Problem/Needs Statement: Reduce the notable health disparities of the target population with emphasis on diabetes management, obesity, cardiovascular disease/hypertension, HIV/AIDS/STDs, and smoking. 42% of adults between ages of 18–44 years live in core target area and 18% of adults are between ages of 45–64 years. The Health Center documents that 35–40% adults (18 to 64 yrs) present for primary care without health insurance.

TABLE E.9

Goals/Objectives	Key Action Steps	Data Source & Evaluation Method	Outcome & Measurement	Person/Area Responsible	Comments
D. Improve adult health between ages of 18 to 44 years.	D.1.(a) Develop marketing strategies and outreach to childbearing aged adults in core target area and extend to catchment area re: access point, TANF requirements and health insurance coverage links.	D.1.(a) Monthly review of outreach activities and linkages with other organizations & employers with adult pops such as Public Welfare Offices, PHA groups.	D.1.(a) 36 sites involved in outreach activities yearly. D.1.(a).1 Marketing materials produced targeting adult interests(health care coverage, health education programs)	D.1.(a) Director, Primary Care Nurse Coordinator, Outreach PHN, Select staff	D.1.(a & b) Established linkage with PA. Adult Basic insurance coverage.
	D.1.(b) Enroll adults in primary care services & refer for case management support for insurance coverage & involve in health education groups.	D.1.(b) Review of client records monthly and case management reports.	D.1.(b) 500 or more adults between 18 & 44 years enroll in care & 25% uninsured apply for health coverage.	D.1.(b) Primary Care Nurse Coordinator, Practice Manager, Social Worker, PHN Case Manager/ Educator	D.1.(b) Health education sessions designed targeting need and interest. Detailed later in Health Plan (obesity, hypertension, exercise, diabetes management).
E. Improve adult health between ages of 45 to 64 years.	E.1.(a) Utilize outreach strategies targeting adult groups with unique needs between ages of 45 & 64 years.	E.1.(a) Monthly review of outreach activities & linkages.	E.1.(a) 36 sites involved in outreach yearly.	E.1.(a) Primary Care Nurse Coordinator, Practice Manager, SW, PHN Case Manager	E.1.(a) Health education sessions regarding adult immunizations, weight control, heart disease, menopause, arthritis available.
	E.1.(b) Enroll adults in primary care services, insurance programs, & involve in health education sessions on-site or in community	E.1.(b) Review of client records monthly, case management reports, health education reports.	E.1.(b) 250 or more adults between ages of 45 & 64 years enroll in care & 20% of uninsured apply for health coverage.	E.1.(b) Primary Care Nurse Coordinator, SW, PHN Case Manager	

Problem/Needs Statement: Census 2000 data indicate that _____ has a significant aging population over 65 years. In the core target area, 16.5% of the population is 65 years and above as compared to citywide elderly population of 13.5%. Aging groups experience increase in chronic diseases and need ongoing disease management to improve quality of life and independent living status.

TABLE E.10

Goals/Objectives	Key Action Steps	Data Source & Evaluation Method	Outcome & Measurement	Person/Area Responsible	Comments
F. Improve health and disparities in disease management of people 65 years and above.	F.1.(a) Develop specific outreach strategies to inform seniors in new access point.	F.1.(a, b, c) Monthly review of outreach activities designed with seniors of diverse cultures, access points, educational and economic levels in mind.	F.1.(a,b,c) 36 sites yearly involved in senior citizen outreach with at least 12 PCA sites involving 1,000 or more senior citizens.	F.1.(a,b,c). Director, Primary Care Clinical Coordinator, Outreach PHN	F.1.(a,b,c) Have established relationships with seniors in public housing units for focus group work, in-place health education contract with PCA, and will incorporate information in program regarding access points available to seniors in their neighborhood.
	F.1.(b) Use public housing focus groups to determine outreach to seniors or soon-to-be seniors in public housing complexes.				
	F.1.(c) Market new access point to seniors involved in _____ Corporation for the Aging (PCA) programs.	F.1.(c) Quarterly review of outreach to seniors involved in PCA programs in catchment area.			
	F.2.(a) Enroll people 65 years of age and above in primary health care services with emphasis on adult influenza vaccines & podiatric care.	F.2.(a) Review of client records for 65 years and above, ascertain level of need, primary care interventions, referrals, linkages with PCA services & other community resources.	F.2.(a) Increase by 3% of people over 65 enrolled at Health Center site.	F.2.(a) Primary Care Clinical Coordinator and staff	F.2.(a) Offer health education programs that address needs and interests of unique senior populations such as public housing residents, Asian groups.

Problem/Needs Statement: The obesity rate of the target population is 28 as compared to citywide index rate of 21. Random record review of 200 enrolled Health Center clients revealed that 43% of clients are obese.

TABLE E.11

Goals/Objectives	Key Action Steps	Data Source & Evaluation Method	Outcome & Measurement	Person/Area Responsible	Comments
G. Reduce health disparities among at-risk target populations through health education, screening initiatives and case management.	G.1.(a) Put in place culturally appropriate services that engage target populations in health education and related screenings programs.	G.1.(a) Monthly review of health education and screening services provided to at-risk groups.	G.1.(a) 12 or more community education and screenings provided yearly & scheduled on-site screenings quarterly (hypertension, stroke, diabetes).	G.1.(a) Director, Outreach PHN, and select staff	G.1.(a) Community linkages in place to provide health education at _____ Center (Korean), Indochinese American Council (Asian, African American), and others.
	G.1.(b) Identify youth with inadequate nutrition—overweight or underweight.	G.1.(b,c,d,e) Quarterly review of community screening data and client records.	G.1.(b) 100 youth identified with inadequate nutrition and counseled/ classes on site.	G.1.(b,c,d,e) Primary Care Nurse Coordinator Outreach PHN, PHN Case Manager, SW	
	G.1.(c) Identify adults and seniors with inadequate nutrition—underweight or overweight.	G.1.(c) Quarterly review of community screening data, client records, & PCA feedback.	G.1.(c) 125 adults identified at risk for inadequate nutrition, counseled, classes on site.		
	G.1.(d) Identify individuals with at-risk or dx with diabetes.	G.1.(d,e) Monthly review of client records and referrals made as indicated.	G.1.(d) 80 or more clients identified at risk for or with diabetes. 90% will have quarterly Hemoglobin A1C screens, annual eye exams, urine tests, and skin integrity exams. ADA standards.		G.1.(d) Clients have on-site counseling, individual and small group through School of Nursing nutrition faculty & students & Diabetes Education Counselor.
	G.1.(e) Identify individuals at risk or dx of hypertension.		G.1.(e) 150 clients identified & 90% have controlled hypertension according to nationally approved standards.		G.1.(d,e) SW will assess clients regarding medication need.

Problem/Needs Statement: Reduce notable childhood health disparities that contribute to premature disability and death. All housing in the target area was built before 1960 including public housing complexes. 24% of children under age 5 years tested positive for lead toxicity. 16.6% of children have asthma. 37.4% of poor children have allergies. 34.2% of children live in household with smoker. Public housing reports housing units have lead and asbestos.

TABLE E.12

Goals/Objectives	Key Action Steps	Data Source & Evaluation Method	Outcome & Measurement	Person/Area Responsible	Comments
H. Reduce impact of environmental health risks to target populations that contribute to chronic diseases such as asthma, lead poisoning, radon, and other topical areas.	H.1.(a) Develop & implement smoking-cessation programs for youth & adults on site and in community settings.	H.1.(a) Program participation & client feedback responses post session, 6 months.	H.1.(a) Four smoking-cessation programs held per year. Minimum of 10 participants per program.	H.1.(a) Outreach PHN, Primary Care Nurse Coordinator, and select staff	H.1.(a) In place smoking-cessation programs on site.
			H.1.(a).1 100 clients or more counseled re: smoking risks & available programs.	H.1.(a).1 Nurse Practitioners, Outreach PHN	
H.1.(b) Implement "Open Airways" asthma education and case management sessions in local schools & homes.	H.1.(b) Review of student participation, feedback and School Nurse reports.	H.1.(b) 120 children in 4 schools participate in Open Airways sessions and 20% have in-home assessments.	H.1.(b) Outreach PHN	H.1.(b) Staff has received "Open Airways" training from American Lung Association	
	H.1.(c) Implement lead screening and education programs with targeted children & caregivers.	H.1.(c) Review of participation in screening programs & lead test results.	H.1.(c) 120 screened in community site, caregivers notified of results, referred as needed.	H.1.(c) Outreach PHN	
	H.1.(d) Provide lead screening tests at access point during regular checkups and other sessions per community indices.	H.1.(d) Review of screening results and follow-up necessary.	H.1.(d) 200 or more children screened on-site for lead exposure & follow-up provided.	H.1.(d) Primary Care Nurse Coordinator, Nurse Practitioners, Medical Assistants	

Problem/Needs Statement: The Housing Authority reports that children in housing units are under-immunized. School nurses report children are not fully immunized and face school expulsion in the target area. Community demand for adult influenza vaccination during Fall 2001 post-September 11 was notable by Center staff; 450 people were immunized in 2001 and 800 adults were immunized in Fall 2002.

TABLE E.13

Goals/Objectives	Key Action Steps	Data Source & Evaluation Method	Outcome & Measurement	Person/Area Responsible	Comments
I. Increase rate of childhood and adult immunizations in target population.	I.1.(a) Conduct infant, children, youth outreach and education programs in catchment area with particular focus on public housing population and émigrés new to area.	I.1. (a) Review monthly of programs and target population engaged with caregivers, school personnel, or staff from other community organizations.	I.1.(a) 1,000 children reached through 12 or more programs. I.1(a).1 500 children reached through 6 programs or more at PHA sites.	I.1.(a) Outreach PHN, Practice Manager	I.1.(a) In-place Immunization Outreach Program funded by City of _____ is an additional resource.
	I.1.(b) Implement childhood immunization campaigns with on-site inoculations provided.	I.1.(b) Review of client records and follow-up date regarding completion of immunizations & School Nurse reports regarding school attendance.	I.1.(b) 350 children will be up to date on immunizations by end of Year 1, 450 by end of Year 2.	I.1.(b) Primary Care Nurse Coordinator, Nurse Practitioners, Medical Assistants, Outreach PHN & select staff	
	I.1.(c) Conduct influenza campaigns targeting adults and chronically ill in local schools, senior centers, and on site in Fall of each year.	I.1.(c) Review of client records post-campaign schedule.	I.1.(c) 500 adults will be immunized in Fall 2002 and another 500 in Fall 2003.	I.1.(c) Primary Care Nurse Coordinator, Nurse Practitioner, Medical Assistants, Outreach PHN & designated staff	

Problem/Needs Statement: To prevent increase in public health threats to target population in catchment area and further urban decline. The public housing populations in zip code 19120 and community residents in adjacent areas (zip codes 19111, 19138, 19141, 19149) represent medically underserved culturally and ethnically diverse groups. The target population lives in declining urban neighborhoods and faces significant disparities in access to quality primary health care services.

TABLE E.14

Goals/Objectives	Key Action Steps	Data Source & Evaluation Method	Outcome & Measurement	Person/Area Responsible	Comments
J. Develop innovative and timely intervention strategies for disadvantaged populations through ongoing monitoring of public housing and community-wide data including health, social, educational, environmental indices that indicate barriers to accessible, affordable, available high-quality primary health care at the new access point.	J.1.(a) Participate in local public housing forums that examine critical health issues of residents.	J.1.(a) Quarterly review of staff contributions to public housing forums.	J.1.(a) 4 or more meetings attended by one or more staff per year.	J.1.(a,b) Director, Practice Manager, Primary Care Nurse Coordinator, PHNs, SW	J.1.(a) The Center is founding member of National Nursing Centers Consortium.
	J.1.(b) Contribute to regional conferences regarding access and urban health needs of underserved culturally diverse groups.	J.1.(b) Quarterly review of participation in regional conferences held by HRSA BPHC, DON and others.	J.1.(b) 2 or more meetings attended by one or more staff per year.		J.1.(b) Director is member of Forum for Primary Health Care. J.1.(b).1 Professional staff belong to professional organizations such as the American Public Health Association, PA Public Health Association, National Association of Nurse Practitioners and others.
	J.1.(c) Share new access point findings and lessons learned in national forums examining the needs and interests of public housing residents.	J.1.(c) Quarterly review of on-site staff meetings and clinical conferences regarding quality improvement measures and presenting primary care needs of clients with attendance logs.	J.1.(c) 100% of staff participate in 3 of 4 quarterly staff meetings held and 95% of health center staff participate in monthly staff meetings on site.	J.1.(c) Director and all staff	
	J.1.(d) Submit report on new access point programs and clinical outcomes.	J.1.(d) Annual report submitted to HRSA BPHC with prior Community Board review.	J.1.(d) Three or more members of team write and submit annual report.	J.1.(d) Director, Practice Manager, Primary Care Nurse Coordinator	

APPENDIX F

Sample Business Plan
(taken from a 330 FQHC
Project Renewal Grant)

TABLE F.1

Health Center

Business Plan for Project Renewal—May 2003

GOVERNANCE:

Problem/Needs Statement: Oversight of RHD Board to HCN Advisory Board needs to be better documented.

Goal/Objective	Key Action Steps	Data Source/ Evaluation Methods	Outcome and Measurement	Person/Area Responsible
A. Provide better mechanism for consumer input to governing Board from the Health Center Advisory Board.	**A.1.** Twice a year, provide a formalized report from the Health Center Advisory Board to the governing board on all HC Advisory Board activity and specifically consumer input.	**A.1.** HC Advisory Board reports.		**A.1.** HC Director, Governing Board Point Person
	A.2. Governing Board Point Person will continue to provide the link to the governing Board by attending all HC Advisory Board Meetings as well as governing board meetings.	**A.2.** Governing Board meeting minutes will reflect input from HC Advisory Board meetings.		**A.2.** Governing Board Point Person

PROGRESS ON PREVIOUS GOALS:

1. **Ensure full representation in the Governance of the Health Center and its activities and meet the requirements of the 330i grant.** The current Health Center Advisory Board was expanded to include community members from the new site—funded through the New Access Point grant in July 2002. Board members received training and orientation along with a copy of the Health Center Advisory Board manual.

TABLE F.2

ADMINISTRATION:

Problems/Need Statement: Network infrastructure needs improvements to better manage overall growth of business operations.

Goal/Objective	Key Action Steps	Data Source/ Evaluation Methods	Outcome/ Measurement	Person/Area Responsible
A. Review/Revise Personnel and Accounting Policies & Procedures.	**A.1.** The current corporate policies and procedures, and the health center specific policy and procedures, will be compared with those provided by the PCER team. Recommendations for changes to either policies will be made by September 30, 2003		**A.1.** Target date September 30, 2003.	**A.1.** HC Financial Director, CFO; HC Business Director
	A.2. A Quality Assurance Plan will be developed based on the finalized accounting policies and procedures by December 31, 2003.	**A.2.** QA Plan will address specific checks & balances and provide for self-audit mechanism.		**A.2.** HC CQI Committee Chairs, HC Advisory Board
B. Revise Affiliation agreement with _____ University to reflect needed safeguards.	**B.1.** Review/Revise Affiliation agreement with University to more clearly state that (a) patient and patient records are the property/responsibility of HC, (b) University personnel are professional contract staff only and compensated for a set amount each month, (c) University clinical staff will follow the clinical protocols of HC and participate in HC's QA program, (d) the property address is listed as the facility where services will be rendered, (e) all federal interests invested in HC as a FQHC are safeguarded and protected.	**B.1.** The revised agreement will be presented to the HC advisory board and the governing board in the Fall, 2003.	**B.1.** BPHC and Advisory Board Approval.	**B.1.** Counsel, HC Director, University Counsel

(continued)

Goal/Objective	Key Action Steps	Data Source/ Evaluation Methods	Outcome/ Measurement	Person/Area Responsible
C. The organizational structure of the health center program will be revised to clarify and better stratify responsibilities and reporting requirements.	**C.1.** The organizational structure of the HC has been discussed and revised at a recent meeting of the HCN management team.	**C.1.** A revised organizational chart has already been sent to the BPHC for review.		**C.1.** HC Director
D. The HC Advisory Board will develop a written, strategic plan (that is approved by the Governing Board) to ensure that HRSA/ BPHC program expectations are fulfilled.	**D.1.** A strategic planning retreat is being scheduled for the Fall, 2003. Organizational consultant will facilitate the process.		**D.1.** Written Strategic Plan will be submitted to BPHC.	**D.1.** HC Director, HC Advisory Board

PROGRESS ON PREVIOUS GOALS:

1. **Maintain a supportive environment for staff and increase staff development opportunities.** Total staff at the health center has almost doubled. Bi-annual staff retreats are now being conducted that provide facilitated exercises in team building, co-operation, stress reduction, and developing good personal relationships with co-workers. Staff satisfaction with this new process was 100% in favor of continuing. HC staff have greatly benefited from all of the HRSA/BPHC trainings offered in addition to numerous trainings provided annually on site and through staff development courses. Supervisors now use a specific section of the performance evaluation tool to discuss staff development issues with and get input from staff. Staff satisfaction surveys have been revised and continue to be distributed and analyzed annually by the CQI committee.

TABLE F.3

Health Center

FINANCIAL:

Problem/Needs Statement: To ensure the HC's long-term viability, an effective strategic financial planning process and more detailed documentation of specific procedures are needed to address increased growth issues and future patient needs.

Goal/Objective	Key Action Steps	Data Source/ Evaluation Methods	Outcome and Measurement	Person/Area Responsible
A. Establish an effective strategic financial planning process to identify resources necessary to make improvements to the infrastructure. Define the most appropriate organizational structure and health care delivery model to meet future needs of patients and assure long-term viability.	**A.1.** Newly created position of Financial Director has been filled to provide oversight to Financial planning and operations.			
	A.2. Technical Assistance (TA) from the BPHC has been requested to assist us in developing a strategic financial planning process.			**A.2.** HC Financial Director
	A.3. TA from BPHC has been requested for developing a system of charges based on Relative Value Units (RVUs).	**A.3.** Using a RVU-based system, provide quarterly review of costs by service department to Department heads.	**A.3.** Actual vs. projected income/expenses will balance.	**A.3.** HC Financial Director, Management Team.
	A.4. Determine increased number of target users/visits for primary care and behavioral health to adequately meet productivity goals.	**A.4.** New Financial plan and Electronic Practice Management System (EPMS) reports provided monthly to track new users and visits.	**A.4.** Visits will increase to meet productivity goals set.	**A.4.** Primary Care Director, BH Director, HC Director
B. Provide clear and comprehensive fiscal policies and procedures to reflect actual HC practice and document the complete HC fiscal process.	**B.1.** Work with CFO to develop a more comprehensive fiscal policies and procedures manual, which reflects all fiscal and accounting systems, including accounts payable and fixed assets/ equipment specifically as they relate to the HC.		**B.1.** Target completion date December 31, 2003.	**B.1.** HC Financial Director, Governing Board Point Person, Chief Financial Officer

(continued)

Goal/Objective	Key Action Steps	Data Source/ Evaluation Methods	Outcome and Measurement	Person/Area Responsible
	B.2. Develop and maintain a log to support the accounts payable process and identify obligated project fund balances.	**B.2.** Monthly comparison of log entries and fiscal reports for consistency.	**B.2.** HC log and reports will balance.	**B.2.** HC Financial Director
C. Improve overall viability by maximizing revenue.	**C.1.** Develop new goals through Financial Plan to determine number of users and reimbursable visits needed to produce needed revenue and adjust productivity formulas accordingly.	**C.1.** EPM visit reports will be generated monthly to Department heads for reviewing individual productivity.	**C.1.** Increase number of users/visits as per new Financial Plan to match resources needed.	**C.1.** HC Business Director, HC Financial Director
	C.2. Continue with renovation plans to acquire use of entire building at health center site to expand service capabilities and increase number of visits. (Awaiting PHA building approval.)	**C.2.** Weekly Renovation meetings.	**C.2.** New space provides additional Exam rooms and additional BH therapy rooms to accommodate increased visits.	**C.2.** HC Director, HC Business Director, Property Manager
	C.3. Continue work with Clinical, Outreach and Front Desk staff to ensue that patients are enrolled in appropriate insurance plans and that the HC is maximizing its MCO and patient fee revenue. Fiscal staff will attend HRSA-sponsored Third-Party Reimbursement training.	**C.3.** Reports generated by EPM, financial management and the MCOs.		HC Director, HC Financial Director, HC Business Director
D. Improve overall viability by minimizing expenses.	**D.1.** Freeze new staff hires until number of visits requires additional staffing as per revised productivity formula.	**D.1.** Monthly productivity report review.	**D.1.** Staff will be added when needed based on appropriate increase in visits.	**D.1.** HC Financial Director, HC Director
	D.2. Strive to reduce the **actual** cost per visit below 2003 PPS rate to create surplus reserves.	**D.2.** Monthly review of expense detail by individual departments and reduce where possible.	**D.2.** Cost Report analysis.	**D.1.** HC Financial Director, HC Director

PROGRESS ON PREVIOUS GOALS:

1. **Establish a provider contract with US Healthcare and other commercial plans.** Despite tireless effort on the part of HC staff, NNCC staff and advocates, and community leaders, US Healthcare executives have not yet credential Nurse Practitioners as PCPs. Blue Cross recently began to credential new Certified Registered Nurse Practitioners (CRNPs) under its managed care plans. Applications for credentialing of our new site staff are currently pending approval.
2. **Increase the number of health center users by 45% (UDS Data).** The HC users have increased by approximately 60%—exceeding target expectations.
3. **Improve collection rate of self-pay fees.** Collected fees increased by 64% (Uniform Data Set [UDS] Data). The newly implemented EPM software is expected to further increase this rate.

Health Center

MANAGEMENT INFORMATION SYSTEMS:

Problem/Needs Statement: Implementation of a new Electronic Practice Management system has greatly changed business operations and needs to be documented.

Goal/Objective	Key Action Steps	Data Source/ Evaluation Methods	Outcome and Measurement	Person/Area Responsible
A. Develop a comprehensive MIS policies and procedures (P& P) manual that reflects actual practice.	**A.1.** Create MIS P&P manual reflecting actual practice and HIPAA compliance issues.	**A.1.** Completed P&P Manual.	**A.1.** Submit Manual for Board Approval by December 31, 2003. Annual review will take place for needed updates.	**A.1.** HC Business Director, HC Data Systems Administrator.
	A.2. Include detailed description of specific relationships with NNCC and _____ Foundation relevant to new Data Project.	**A.2.** Completed P&P Manual.		**A.2.** HC Business Director, HC Data Systems Administrator.
B. Become HIPAA Compliant in all relevant areas.	**B.1.** Effective April 14, 2003, HC is compliant with Privacy Notice/Policy requirements.	**B.1.** Signed, dated Acknowledgement forms are obtained for every patient.	**B.1.** QA Chart Audits will be conducted twice a year for compliance.	**B.1.** CQI Committee designees.
	B.2 HC has requested and been granted an extension for compliance with Standard Code Sets. However, the new EPM system recently implemented at the HC is currently HIPAA compliant.	**B.2.** Contract with Misys Healthcare Systems and purchaser, Foundation, Terms of Gift Agreement with HC.		**B.2.** Foundation Data Project Manager
	B.3. Maintain all necessary Business Associate Agreements as required by HIPAA.	**B.3.** All agreements are currently on file.		**B.3.** HC Business Director
	B.4. Improve patient confidentiality at reception desk by including in renovation plans a separate and more private area for patient registration and conversations. At site locations where space does not permit this, reception staff will escort patients to a private room when necessary.	**B.4.** Confidentiality is one of the requested measures on Patient Satisfaction Surveys, which are conducted twice a year.	**B.4.** Patient Satisfaction Survey results will be analyzed by CQI Committee designees twice a year and QA Plans developed as needed to address concerns.	**B.4.** CQI Committee Chairs, HC Business Director, HC Administrative Director

(continued)

TABLE F.4 *(continued)*

Goal/Objective	Key Action Steps	Data Source/ Evaluation Methods	Outcome and Measurement	Person/Area Responsible
	B.5. With the implementation of the new EPM, we have been able to ensure that ALL access to patient information is based on minimum necessary rule by applying security level access. All access is password protected. NNCC Data Administrator has access to log of all user access/activity.	**B.5.** Self-Audit/Spot checks will be conducted at each site re: PC screen locks, chart locations, sign-in privacy.		**B.5.** NNCC Data Administrator, HC Data Systems Administrator, HC Business Director

PROGRESS ON PREVIOUS GOALS:

1. **Improve health outcomes by utilizing the Electronic Medical Record.** EMR implementation has been delayed due to the discontinuance of the software data system. The Network chose to participate in the NNCC Data Project, which included a gift of the Misys Healthcare Systems software for EMR and EPM and allows shared aggregate data amongst all participating health centers. The EPM module (Tiger), which is designed to specifically capture previously missed financial data for FQHCs, was implemented April 1, 2003 at all 3 health center sites and has already improved fiscal operations. Implementation of the EMR module is scheduled to begin in Fall 2003 and will also include all Network sites.

Appendix G

Sample of a Contract with a Local Agency

December 30, 2002

RE: Contractual Engagement for Specific Services Rendered by the Family Health Center of _____ to _____ on behalf of the National Nursing Centers Consortium in regards to the Lead-Safe Babies Project, funded by the U.S. Environmental Protection Agency.

This Contract is to confirm our understanding for _____ as fiscal agent for the National Nursing Centers Consortium (hereinafter referred to as "NNCC") to engage Provider as an independent contractor to perform certain services for the NNCC under the terms and conditions set forth in this Letter of Agreement.

This letter, when signed by the director of the service provider and returned to the NNCC, will constitute an agreement with the intention of being legally binding as follows:

1. Fiscal Agent hereby engages Provider as a consultant to provide Specific Services on behalf of the NNCC as stated in the attached Scope of Work.
2. The specific services the Provider will perform and the specific schedule for providing these services shall be in accordance with the provisions of Paragraph One (1) and may be as reasonably necessary or appropriate for the program to which it relates.
3. Provider shall perform all services under this Letter of Agreement in accordance with all applicable laws, regulations, other governing rule and standards, and the requirements of the program to which it relates, and shall perform all services in a manner consistent and in compliance with all

accepted and prevailing standards for the proper performance of the same or similar services. The period of this contract shall be from September 1, 2002 to March 31, 2004; and may be terminated by either party with 3-day written notification to the other party, without cause or liability other than to compensate for services performed to the date of termination.

4. Subject to the availability of funds for this purpose, and in consideration of the specific services performed by Provider, and upon receipt of invoice and subsequent approval by Fiscal Agent under this Agreement, the NNCC shall pay a provider service fee of $50 up to 20 target clients, or 40 visits; this fee includes reimbursement for expenses incurred in the course of performing the above services. Work will be scheduled upon mutual agreement between the Provider and the NNCC.
5. Provider warrants that the performance will be of the highest professional quality.
6. Provider shall indemnify, defend, and hold harmless the NNCC/Fiscal Agent from and against any and all losses, claims, actions, damages, liability, and expenses, including reasonable attorneys' fees incurred by the NNCC in connection with, arising out of, or resulting from any act or omission of Provider's agent, contractors, or servants pursuant to this contract.
7. NNCC/Fiscal Agent shall indemnify, defend, and hold harmless Provider from and against any and all loses, claims, actions, damages, liability and expenses, including reasonable attorney's fees incurred by Provider in connection with, arising out of, or resulting from any act or omission of the NNCC's/Fiscal Agent's agents, contractors, employees, or servants pursuant to this contract.

8. The NNCC shall own all rights in and to the services provided, including copyrights and patents. Service Provider agrees to execute any documents that may be necessary to protect the NNCC's/Fiscal Agent's ownership rights.

9. Provider's relationship to the NNCC shall be one of independent contractor. Provider shall not in any manner be deemed an agent or employee of the NNCC/Fiscal Agent, and shall have no authority to bind or obligate, or incur any liability on behalf of the NNCC/Fiscal Agent, and no such authority shall be implied.

10. Pennsylvania law shall govern the validity, construction, interpretation, and effect of this Letter of Agreement.

11. Provider, as an independent contractor, shall obtain and maintain during the term of the Letter of Agreement all required liability insurances to include, if applicable, professional malpractice liability insurance for the services provided under this Letter of Agreement and make every effort to name Fiscal Agent/NNCC as an additional insured under such policy.

Indicate your acceptance of the terms of the Letter of Agreement by signing in the space provided below. Please return a signed copy of this Letter of Agreement to Fiscal Agent. This Letter shall not be binding unless and until NNCC receives a copy duly executed by you. Thank you.

_____

_____
Date

SCOPE OF WORK: LEAD-SAFE BABIES PROVIDER

ENVIRONMENTAL PROTECTION AGENCY, REGION III NATIONAL NURSING CENTERS CONSORTIUM (NNCC)

Organizational Overview:

The National Nursing Centers Consortium (NNCC) was established in 1996, and is an association of nurse-managed community health centers in the U.S.

Relationship of Provider to NNCC:

The Provider, an identified partner in the grant, is a member nurse-managed health center of the National Nursing Centers Consortium. In an effort to foster the growth and sustainability of the nursing centers, the NNCC contracts with its centers to perform outreach and education of the community. Stipends for reimbursement are based on time allocated to project and cost needs of the center.

Proposed Intervention:

Educational home and hospital visits to women in their last trimester of pregnancy and mothers with newborn children up to 6 months of age.

Method/Target Areas:

Pregnant women and new mothers that live in the rural Pennsylvania target area of Greene county. Referrals will be made by area nursing centers. Women can also refer themselves to the program, which will be advertised through posters and brochures.

Intervention/Statement of Work:

Outreach workers from the Provider will be responsible for the recruitment of clients from hospitals, community health centers, and clients of the nurse-managed health center. Referral/Intake information will be taken by staff at the nurse-managed health center and recorded in a program database. Upon receipt of the referral information, outreach workers will conduct introductory visits for up to 20 clients. Between 180 and 210 days later, a follow-up visit will be conducted; if the follow-up visit is not conducted within the designated timeframe, reimbursement will be lost. The visits will consist of in-house presentations and information on lead poisoning prevention techniques. Emphasis will be placed on actions the caregiver can us, such as hand washing, cleaning techniques, and proper nutrition. A short pre-test will be administered to the caregiver to ascertain her level of knowledge about lead. Participants will be provided with incentives, including a "lead bucket" filled with supplies to enable them to clean the lead dust, e.g., sponges, detergent, and hand soap. The healthcare worker will also teach the caregiver the appropriate way to avoid lead poisoning and present literature for the caregiver to keep. The follow-up visit will begin with the administration of a post-test, to measure retained knowledge about lead. During the visit, the outreach worker will review lead poisoning prevention techniques discussed in the first visit. At the end of the visit, the outreach worker will present the caregiver with a gift card.

Target Audience:

Primary prevention geared toward 100 pregnant women and new mothers living in the following target counties of rural Pennsylvania: Allegheny, Greene, Huntingdon, Montgomery, and Northumberland.

Time Period of Program:

September 30, 2002—March 31, 2002
During the grant period, the partners will meet regularly to review activities, report progress and problems, report client feedback, and correct problems. In order to ensure that the program meets its goals and objective the NNCC will track the:

1. Number of lead education visits;
2. Number of families lost to follow up;
3. Increase in baseline knowledge, attitudes, and behaviors regarding lead poising on the part of program clients;
4. Lead levels of children screened.

APPENDIX H

Funding Sources

GOVERNMENT

Federal Grants:

Bureau of Primary Health Care/Health Resources and Services Administration
http://bphc.hrsa.gov/Grants/Default.htm

Centers for Disease Control
http://www.cdc.gov/funding.htm

Substance Abuse and Mental Health Services Administration
http://www.samhsa.gov/grants/grants.html

U.S. Department of Health and Human Services
http://www.dhhs.gov/grants/index.shtml
http://www.dhhs.gov/grantsnet/grantinfo.htm

State Grants:

State's Department of Public Health

City/Local Grants:

City's Department of Public Health

FOUNDATIONS

The Annenberg Foundation
http://www.whannenberg.org
Purpose: Support primarily for early childhood and K–12 education (including public school restructuring and re-form). Some support for cultural programs and health education.

The Annie E. Casey Foundation
http://www.aecf.org/
Purpose: The primary mission is to foster public policies, human service reforms, and community supports that more effectively meet the needs of vulnerable families and children.

The Commonwealth Fund
http://www.cmwf.org
Purpose: The four major program areas are international health care policy and practice, improving the quality of health care services, improving insurance coverage and access to care, and improving public spaces and services.

Bill & Melinda Gates Foundation
http://www.gatesfoundation.org/
Purpose: The foundation favors preventive approaches and collaborative endeavors with government, philanthropic, and not-for-profit partners. Priority is given to grants that leverage additional support and serve as a catalyst for long-term, systemic change.

Helene Fuld Trust
http://www.fuldtrust.org
Purpose: Leadership development for nursing students, educational mobility, and curriculum and faculty development in community-based care.

The Pew Charitable Trusts
http://www.pewtrusts.com
Purpose: The health and human services program should be designed to promote the health and well-being of the American people and to strengthen disadvantaged communities.

Pfizer Foundation

http://www.pfizer.com/subsites/philanthropy/inde x.html
Purpose: The foundation provides grants targeted at health care and the sciences. Specifically, in terms of community and cultural programs, Pfizer focuses on those in the New York area because it is home to Pfizer's global headquarters. Organizations in communities beyond the New York headquarters should contact the community relations or public relations representative at the site about submitting a proposal.

Public Welfare Foundation

http://www.publicwelfare.org
Purpose: This non-governmental grant-making organization supports organizations that provide services to disadvantaged populations and work for lasting improvements in the delivery of services that meet basic human needs. An initial request should come in the form of a letter of inquiry. The foundation has provided grants in the following areas: criminal justice, disadvantaged elderly and youth, environment, population, health, community and economic development, human rights and technology assistance.

Robert Wood Johnson Foundation

http://www.rwjf.org
Purpose: The foundation is devoted exclusively to health and health care and concentrates its grantmaking in three areas: assuring access to basic health services for all Americans at reasonable cost; improving the way services are organized and provided for people with chronic health conditions; and reducing the harm caused by substance abuse—tobacco, alcohol, and illicit drugs.

W. K. Kellogg Foundation

http://www.wkkf.org
Purpose: The goal of the foundation's health program is to improve the health of people in communities through increased access to integrated, comprehensive health care systems that are organized around public health, prevention, and primary health care, and that are guided, managed, and staffed by a wide range of appropriately prepared personnel.

Washington Square Health Foundation

http://www.wshf.org
Purpose: Giving to organizations, primarily in the Chicago area, that provide significant health-related benefits. Eligible categories include health services, medical research, or medical education.

APPENDIX I

Sample Policy and Procedure Manual

FAMILY PRACTICE AND COUNSELING NETWORK POLICIES AND PROCEDURES MANUAL

The following is a prototype of policies that one should include in their policy and procedure manual.

GENERAL POLICIES AND PROCEDURES

1. INTRODUCTION:
   Mission Statement
   History and Services
   Organization Chart

2. EMPLOYEE BENEFITS:
   See RHD Corporate Human Resources Policies
   Network Salary and Other Compensation
   Behavioral Health Treatment Limitations for Network Staff
   Network Employees Paid Time Off—Full-Time
   Network Employees Paid Time Off—Part-Time

3. WORK CONDITIONS AND ENVIRONMENT:
   Management Team Operations
   Staff Meetings
   Policies and Procedures
   Staff Recruitment and Retention
   Professional Liability
   Credentialing
   Continuing Education
   Adding Clinical Staff
   Productivity Standards
   Performance Evaluations
   Safety and Accident Prevention
   Infection Control
   Vehicle Safety
   See RHD Policy #503—Smoking, Safety, and Handling Bodily Fluids
   See RHD Policy #504—Accidents and Injuries
   Maintaining Office Space
   Office Closing
   Night Closing
   Staff Travel Reimbursement

4. URGENT/EMERGENCY SITUATIONS:
   Crisis Management
   Code Blue
   Hospitalization
   Incident Reporting

5. EMPLOYEE CONDUCT:
   RHD Bill of Rights and Responsibilities for Employees and Consumers
   See RHD Policy #602—Employee Rules of Conduct
   See RHD Policy #610—Dispute Resolution
   Network Code of Conduct
   Network Conflict Resolution Policy
   Confidentiality
   RHD HIPAA Privacy Policy
   RHD HIPAA Privacy Procedures
   Child Abuse Reporting
   Elder Abuse Reporting
   Cultural Competence
   Dress Code
   HIPAA Short Form

6. PATIENTS' RIGHTS:
   Network Patients' Rights
   Behavioral Health Civil Rights
   Consent for Treatment
   Parental Consent for Minors
   Services for Patients with Limited English Proficiency and Hearing Impairments

Patient Complaints and Grievances
Behavioral Health Attendance Agreement Form
Civil Rights Compliance Form

7. PROGRAM OPERATIONS:
Appointment Scheduling Standards and Tracking
Hours of Operation
On-Call Coverage
Referral to Outside Providers
Educating Students
Sliding Scale Assessments
Record Completion and Documentation
Pharmaceutical Storage and Handling
Refilling Psychiatric Medications
Physician Consultants for Primary Care

8. CONTINUOUS QUALITY IMPROVEMENT:
Strategic Planning
Quality of Care
Performance Improvement Plan
Internal Chart Audits
Stakeholder Input

9. TRANSPORTATION SUPPORT SERVICES:
A. UTILIZATION:
Eligibility and Authorization for Services
Authorization Form
Scheduling and Tracking of Van Services
Non-Patient Use of the Vans

B. DRIVERS:
Responsibilities of Drivers
Safety Restraint Requirements
Substitute Drivers

C. PASSENGERS:
Responsibilities of Passengers
Passenger Handout

D. VAN MAINTENANCE:
Maintenance and Repair of Vehicles
Vehicle Service Information Form

10. JOB DESCRIPTIONS:

NURSE PRACTITIONER CLINICAL PRACTICE GUIDELINES and BEHAVIORAL HEALTH STANDARDS/POLICIES AND PROCEDURES are two separate manuals not contained in this book.

STAKEHOLDER INPUT

Purpose: The purpose of this policy is to outline the procedure for obtaining input that will contribute to the quality of care from the stakeholders in the Family Practice and Counseling Network.

Policy: The Performance Improvement (PI) Committee will guide the process of obtaining input from the stakeholders in the Network's services. The PI Committee will define who the stakeholders in each service are. Stakeholders fall into three categories: the individuals and families served, the customers/payers, and the communities that the Network serves.

Procedures: Individuals and families served will be surveyed individually to determine their satisfaction with the services they are receiving. A standardized survey instrument that ensures anonymity and allows results to be shared with other nurse-managed centers will be used. All clients will be told upon coming into services that their opinion of services will be sought.

- Random surveys of 100 cases served in each office will be done twice annually. Front desk will give surveys to clients coming in for services. After they are completed, surveys are put into a closed container to assure confidentiality. The National Nursing Center Consortium tabulates patient surveys.
- Another way that satisfaction may be determined is through the use of focus groups. This may be particularly successful with teenagers or people using group services. Surveys may also be used to determine the satisfaction of customers/payers or representatives of the community with the services being provided by the Network. Staff members will also be surveyed.
- The results of stakeholder surveys will be tabulated and the results will be included in the Quality Improvement meetings.

STRATEGIC PLANNING

Purpose: This policy outlines the strategic planning process that the Family Practice and Counseling Network conducts in order to:

- Clarify the mission, values and mandates of the Network;
- Assess the strengths, weaknesses, opportunities and threats of the organization;
- Establish goals and objectives, which flow from the mission and the Network's mandated responsibilities;
- Assess financial and human resources needs; and

- Identify and formulate strategies to meet identified goals.

Policy: At least every 4 years, the Network will conduct a system-wide, long-term strategic planning process. The Management Team will work with the Advisory Board to develop the strategic plan. The process will begin with a strategic analysis, which will include a needs assessment and, using the information gathered in the needs assessment and the ongoing quality improvement process, an analysis of the Network's strengths, weaknesses, opportunities, and threats. Then a Board and Management retreat will be held where the future directions of the Network, including goals, objectives, strategies, and resource needs, will be developed.

The Advisory Board, as well as the Board of RHD, will review the final Strategic Plan and approve it. The Strategic Plan will be part of the Board Manual distributed to all Advisory Board members and will be given to staff members as well.

Procedures: Needs Assessment

An extensive community needs assessment will be conducted that will include demographic information regarding the areas and populations served and will examine trends in the systems in which the Network functions and changes that have taken place or are projected. The needs assessment will include the development of demographic profiles of the community served and of the actual population of persons being served.

The needs assessment will also include surveys of stakeholders—persons served, staff, RHD board and management members, members of the Network's Advisory Board and advisory committees, volunteers, community representatives and contractor organization and referral source staff—to determine:

- Their perceptions of changing community conditions, trends, and needs, particularly in areas that the Network may be able to address; and
- Their opinions of the Network's current performance and what the Network could do to improve services.

SWOT Analysis

The Network will conduct an analysis of its Strengths, Weaknesses, Opportunities, and Threats, using the information gathered in the Quality Improvement process and the needs assessment.

The Advisory Board and as many staff members as possible will be involved in a series of meetings where the SWOT analysis will be conducted. The information generated will be distilled into an integrated analysis that will identify the strategic issues facing the organization, which will be distributed to all of the people who will participate in the planning retreat that will generate the elements of the final Strategic Plan.

Strategic Plan Structure

The Strategic Plan will briefly discuss the reason and process for the development of the Plan and then will consist of three sections: the History, Mission, Population, and Services of the Network; a Strategic Analysis of the Network's Current Position, including the Strategic Issues determined at the retreat; and the Network's Future Directions, including goals and objectives, strategies for achievement, resource requirements, designation of responsibility, and timeframes. An Executive Summary may be included, as well as detailed appendices, which may include:

- Description of Strategic Planning Process—A description of the process used to develop the plan, who was involved, minutes of the retreat, and any major lessons learned to improve planning the next time around.
- Strategic Analysis Data—The detailed information generated during the needs assessment and the SWOT analysis.
- Budget Plan—The detailed description of the resources and funding needed to achieve the strategic goals.
- Health Care Plan—A description of the service goals and activities to be accomplished over the coming year in the format required by HRSA.
- Business Plan—A description of the operational goals and activities to be accomplished over the coming year in the format required by HRSA.
- Quality Improvement Plan—A description of the detailed process for monitoring and improving the services of the Network.

QUALITY OF CARE

Purpose: The purpose of this policy is to outline the Performance Improvement program of the Family Practice and Counseling Network.

Policy: The Family Practice and Counseling Network is committed to providing the highest possible quality of services and to the safety and satisfaction of the people who receive those services. In order to maintain and improve the quality of the health centers' processes and outcomes, in keeping with the Network mission statement, goals, and beliefs, the Network will follow a systematic Performance Improvement Plan for monitoring and evaluating the safety, quality, and appropriateness of patient care and for identifying and resolving problems. (See the Network Performance Improvement Plan.)

Plan: The objectives of the Performance Improvement process are the following:

- The program ensures continued and accessible healthcare by protection and appropriate utilization of resources.
- The program ensures staff, visitor, and patient safety.
- The program ensures the competency of clinical staff.
- The program routinely and systematically monitors indicators of patient satisfaction.

The Board is ultimately responsible for the quality of all phases of center operations. The Executive Director and the Primary Care Network Director provide leadership for accessing and providing data relevant to recognizing opportunities to improve. The Performance Improvement Committee is comprised of leadership members and clinic staff members and has representation from all areas of operations to facilitate an interdisciplinary approach. Staff and professional meetings are held regularly in order to enhance opportunities for all staff to participate in problems identification, solution, and quality improvement. The Performance Improvement Committee meets at least quarterly and the results of these meetings are shared with staff.

The Performance Improvement process works with four types of information:

- Incidents and accidents and grievances, including safety data, such as:
  - Documented sentinel events, incidents, or injuries (see Incident Reporting Policy);
  - Infections that may have been acquired through rendering of care or may be potentially communicable to the community or staff;
  - OSHA in-service trainings, CPR recertifications, fire safety education, and compliance with evacuation procedures; and

- Staff knowledge of disaster procedures and emergency preparedness.

- Record reviews and audits for compliance, resource utilization, and quality issues (see Primary Care Peer Review Procedure and Behavioral Health Internal Chart Audit and Peer Review Procedures);
  - Peer reviews using case reviews in clinical staff meetings and through chart audits;
  - NP meetings with collaborating physicians to review patient records and discuss cases.

- Patient, staff, and other stakeholder input (see stakeholder Input Procedure); and
- Clinical care and service indicators and outcomes data, including:
  - Statistical data reviewed for trends and changes in population demographics and needs for services that may impact future planning;
  - Clinical care measures of service outcomes that are dictated by the Network Health Care Plan; and
  - Appointment compliance and continuity of care data.

The review of QI information may result in the development and implementation of performance improvement studies, which include the following steps:

- Opportunity/problem identification,
- Development of criteria,
- Data collection,
- Data analysis,
- Development of an action plan,
- Follow up.

Actions that may be carried out by service units and/ or the QI Committee to achieve Network Performance Improvement objectives include:

- Regular credentialing of all clinicians;
- Enhancing staff satisfaction by fostering the growth and development of all staff;
- Annual review and updating of evidence-based policies and procedures in the Clinical Standards of Care Manuals for all Primary Care Providers;
- Providing regular forums for clinicians to discuss and review clinical issues and cases among themselves and with collaborating physicians.

Individual patient and staff confidentiality is respected within the evaluation and reporting of Performance Improvement activities. Although information regarding Performance Improvement activities is available to internal and external consumers, minutes of meetings and raw data are not discoverable outside the organization without prior approval of the Board. The Network may participate in data warehousing with other health centers but the data is de-identified of specific patient information to observe and protect individual's privacy. The Network complies with the latest HIPAA guidelines regarding patient information.

INTERNAL CHART AUDITS

Purpose: The purpose of this policy is to outline the procedure for performing monthly chart audits in order to assure accuracy, timeliness in the billing and collection of fees for service, and quality of care and appropriateness of outcomes.

Policy: An internal chart audit will be performed on a monthly basis. The audit will be conducted on services that occurred 6 months prior in order to allow for the billing, payment, rejection, and rebilling process to be completed.

In order to assure that a significant sample of records is reviewed, at least ten records from each site will be reviewed each month. If problems are found, a higher number of cases may be reviewed. Also, if some kinds of cases are identified as high-risk or problem-prone, a higher percentage of those kinds of cases will be reviewed.

All clinical staff will participate in reviews and will review records within their own discipline. However, no reviewer will review any cases in which they have been directly involved or involved in a supervisory capacity. All professional disciplines involved in a service will be represented in the peer review process for that service. All peer reviewers will receive training in the review process.

The results of the record reviews will tabulated from the review forms. The results will be included in each quarterly Quality Improvement meeting.

Procedure: The following steps will be followed:

1. Randomly select 5% or 5 (whichever is greater) patients who had visits from the Hours Report.
2. Obtain and review the following documents:
   a. Patient's chart,
   b. Single Event Report (SER) where patient's service is recorded by clinician,
   c. Invoice for patient's service,
   d. Remittance advice where service was paid,
   e. Authorization if applicable,
   f. Rejection notice if applicable.
3. Complete the Internal Chart Audit Form, noting any discrepancies between what was billed and what was recorded in the chart.
4. If there are any discrepancies, determine and record the Corrective Action required to correct that discrepancy and to avoid repeating the same discrepancy in the future.
5. Determine and record the timeframe necessary to complete the Corrective Action.
6. Obtain signature and date from Behavioral Health Director.

APPOINTMENT SCHEDULING STANDARDS AND TRACKING PROCEDURES

Purpose: The purpose of this policy is to detail the proper protocol for scheduling and tracking appointments.

Policy: The Network Health Centers are committed to providing appointments to patient within a reasonable period of time, depending on the severity of the problem. The appointment system is flexible to allow for accommodating emergencies. Priority is placed on urgent "walk-ins" and on scheduled appointments. Patients who walk in without an appointment, and who do not have an urgent problem, are accommodated in the most timely fashion possible. Each health center provides hours that meet accessibility needs of the community served.

Below each type of appointment is defined and a standard timeframe for offering an appointment is specified.*

When in doubt about determining the urgency of ANY appointment, the Receptionist or Medical Assistant will rely on the judgment of the clinician to determine the urgency of a presented problem.

I. Scheduling Standards:

A. Primary Care

1. **Emergency Problem**—An emergency is defined as one that without immediate medical attention

---

*All centers operate under an open access policy, which attempts to schedule patients the same day or next business day regardless of the reason for the appointment.

would likely cause the patient to suffer serious harm or deterioration.

Examples—Heavy bleeding of a laceration or wound, asthma attack or other respiratory distress, severe chest pain, or anyone who appears to be in severe physical or psychological distress.

Standard: This person receives immediate attention/triage and is given priority over other patients who do not have emergent problems.

2. **Urgent Problem**—An urgent problem is one that requires prompt attention but is not a medical emergency.

    Examples—Examples of urgent problems are fever, earaches, abdominal pains, sprains, and strains. It is a new acute problem, or an ongoing problem that has very recently deteriorated or become acute.

    Standard: Same day or next business day appointment is offered. Some problems must be seen the same day, such as a new injury that may be a fracture or a very high fever, earache, or severe pain.

3. **Routine Appointment**—A routine appointment is one where there is no acute illness.

    Examples—Regular family planning visits, well child/adolescent/adult visits, follow-up on a chronic or ongoing problem.

    Standard: Patients will be offered a choice of at least two appointment times the same day or next business day within a maximum of 10 business days of the request.

4. **Prenatal Appointment**—All appointments during a patient's pregnancy.

    Standard: Appointment is offered within 10 business days of request.

5. **Family Planning Emergencies**—A request for pregnancy testing or emergency contraceptives.

    Standard: Pregnancy Testing—Appointment will be scheduled the same day or next business day.

    Emergency Contraceptives—Appointment will attempt to be scheduled the same day or next business day but no longer than 72 hours after unprotected sex.

B. Behavioral Health

1. **Standard Appointments**

    Current Patients—Appointments will be scheduled by the treating clinician and/or department assistant at a frequency and time agreed upon by the patient and the clinician.

New Patients—A patient is called within 2 business days of the initial referral. Assessment appointment will be scheduled within 5 business days of making the contact with the patient, OR the patient will be provided with referrals to alternative site(s) for treatment. Patient can request to be on Behavioral Health waiting list.

2. **Urgent Appointments**

    Current Patients—For a current patient, an urgent appointment will be scheduled as soon as the treating clinician has an opening or within 24 hours by any available clinician, whichever the patient prefers.

    New Patients—A new patient will be seen within 24 hours or referred elsewhere for urgent care.

3. **Emergency Appointments**

    Current Patients—A current patient needing emergency care will be responded to immediately during business hours, and within 30 minutes by the on-call clinician when the health center is closed.

    New Patients—Emergency appointments are provided for new patients within 1 hour if there is a clinician available at the time the emergency presents. Otherwise, emergent patients will be referred and/or transported to the nearest ER, CRC or other facility equipped to handle emergencies.

II. Tracking Procedures:

A. Primary Care

No-Show:

Front desk staff notifies patients of their appointment at least 1 day ahead of time. Charts of patients who miss an appointment are referred to an NP who determines appropriate follow-up within 24 hours of the missed appointment. Patients who are considered to be vulnerable are referred to the appropriate person for care/case management. Patients who repeatedly miss appointments may be double-booked for future appointments.

Late Arrival:

Patients arriving more than 15 minutes past the scheduled appointment time will be treated as a "Walk-In." The patient also has the option of re-scheduling their appointment for another available time slot within a 2-week period.

Exceptions to this policy may be made for emergencies—as determined by a Nurse Practitioner.

When being asked to reschedule an appointment due to lateness, the patient will be treated in a polite and nonjudgmental manner.

B. Behavioral Health

No-Show:

1. **For clients being seen for the first time:**
   a. The client is scheduled for an appointment and given a courtesy call prior to the appointment (either the day before or the morning of the appointment) to be reminded of the time he/she is expected to meet with the therapist.
   b. Clients who miss appointments without canceling are contacted by phone to reschedule the appointment. At that time, it is explained that another "no-show" will result in a conversation outlining whether or not the individual is ready for therapy at this time.
   c. If a new client misses an Intake appointment for the third time, no further attempts to schedule an appointment are made. A phone call is made or a letter issued asking the client to contact the office if interested in therapy at a later date. However, the client is asked to wait at least 30 days before rescheduling. A client may also be referred elsewhere for appropriate services.

2. **For clients who are currently in treatment:**
   Missing an appointment without calling to cancel is not acceptable. All clients are informed of the importance of keeping appointments and asked to sign a written statement of the following attendance policy, which is kept on file:
   a. If a client misses three consecutive appointments without canceling at least 24 hours in advance, the case is closed. The client is asked to wait at least 60 days before trying to re-engage services.
   b. After the second consecutive missed appointment without sufficient notice, the client is reminded of this policy and given a reminder that a third consecutive "no-show" will result in closure of the case.
   c. If the client's case has been closed, new assessment procedures must be completed to re-open the case and re-engage in treatment.
   d. Patients who chronically no-show may be booked for a 30-minute session at the same time as another patient who is a chronic no-

show patient. The person who shows up first is seen for the first half hour. If both patients show up, they each get a 30-minute visit. If only one patient shows up, they receive a full 45-minute session.

3. **Exceptions:**
   Exceptions to this policy may be made on a case-by-case basis. We will always endeavor to assist clients in serious crisis to obtain appropriate services (e.g., client is suicidal, homicidal, or in imminent need of hospitalization).

Late Arrival:

1. If a patient is more than 30 minutes late for a therapy appointment, one of the following may occur:
   a. The patient may be seen for the remainder of the scheduled time.
   b. The patient may be rescheduled and a "no-show" recorded for the appointment.
2. If a patient is more than 10 minutes late for a psychiatric appointment (medication check or Psychiatric Evaluation) or for an Intake Assessment, one of the following may occur:
   a. The patient may be seen for the remainder of the scheduled time.
   b. The patient may be rescheduled and a "no-show" recorded for the appointment.

Exceptions to this policy may be made on a case-by-case basis—as determined by a Behavioral Health clinician.

When being asked to reschedule an appointment due to lateness, the patient will be treated in a polite and nonjudgmental manner.

PHYSICIAN CONSULTANTS FOR PRIMARY CARE

Purpose: The purpose of this policy is to describe the role of the physician consultant as required by Pennsylvania State Rules and Regulations.

Policy: The Network contracts with physicians who act as collaborators with the Nurse Practitioners. The physicians' role is to actively consult with the Nurse Practitioners regarding patient care and the prescribing of medications.

The Nurse Practitioners use agreed-upon standards of care and clinical practice guidelines. These guidelines are maintained in a separate manual.

Physician(s) provide on-site consultation at regular intervals as is required to meet the needs of the Practice. On these visits, they may review medical charts, discuss protocols and standards of care, or see a patient. There is a physician collaborating agreement for each Nurse Practitioner, which is signed by both parties and kept on file in the health center. These agreements are approved by the State Board of Nursing and allow Nurse Practitioners to sign prescriptions according to formularies.

ON-CALL AND EMERGENCY POLICY

Purpose: The purpose of this policy is to describe the procedure for providing continuous care to Network patients when the health centers are closed.

Policy: It is both a necessity for quality care and a requirement of managed care organizations that patients have access to a Primary Care Provider at all times.

Procedures:

Primary Care:

The Health Centers maintain Primary Care hours daily Monday through Friday and, in two of the sites, two (2) Saturdays a month. The hours at each center are determined to meet the needs of the communities served and are re-evaluated and adjusted as needed.

After hours, a Nurse Practitioner is always on-call to respond to urgent matters. All calls are returned by the Nurse Practitioner on call within 30 minutes of receiving a page. Patients are assessed by phone and are advised appropriately. If necessary, a patient is referred to the nearest emergency room. If indicated, a direct call is made to the emergency room to facilitate emergency care for the patient.

It is the responsibility of the front desk staff to assure that telephones are set at the close of business each day to forward calls appropriately to the answering service.

Behavioral Health:

All clients are informed of on-call services at Intake. Clients are given a card at Intake with the phone numbers to call for after-hours assistance.

The Behavioral Health department maintains hours Monday through Friday in at least one of the health center locations. The hours are determined to meet the needs of the communities served and are re-evaluated and adjusted as needed.

After hours, a Behavioral Health clinician is always on call to respond to urgent matters involving current patients.

Callers who are not current patients of our Behavioral Health service may be asked to call back during business hours or redirected to city emergency services.

The clinician on call returns all calls within 30 minutes of receiving a page. Patients are assessed by phone and are advised appropriately. If necessary, a patient is referred to an emergency room or crisis response center. If indicated, a direct call is made to the emergency room to facilitate emergency care for the patient. Mobile Crisis services or emergency services may also be dispatched at the judgment of the on-call clinician. Primary Care on-call staff may also be called for assistance.

Every salaried clinician takes a turn being on call. The pager is rotated weekly among available clinicians. The schedule is posted to the answering service and the Primary Care department every 6 months. If a clinician will not be available during a scheduled rotation, it is the responsibility of that clinician to arrange for alternate coverage and to notify the answering service and the Behavioral Health Director of the schedule change.

EDUCATING STUDENTS

Purpose: The purpose of this policy is to describe the health center policy on educating students.

Policy: The Network encourages teaching activities during the regular workday that are in keeping with the health center mission.

The Network is committed to the training of students and post-graduate trainees in a variety of professional fields. The supervising clinician has ultimate responsibility for the work of students.

Each individual from a training program shall be assigned at all times to a supervising clinician. It shall be the responsibility of each such clinician to observe and counsel the trainee on a patient-by-patient basis and to countersign all clinical notes written by the trainee. Prior to a visit with a student, the patient's permission must be obtained. A patient has the right to refuse care by a student. In primary care, the clinician must, during the course of a patient visit by a student, have direct, face-to-face contact with the patient.

In behavioral health, the supervising clinician oversees all care provided by trainees. This oversight may include: direct observation of the trainee, review of audio tapes or verbatim session notes, review of patient charts and all clinical documentation, evaluations, test reports, etc. The supervising clinician will countersign test reports, assessments, treatment plans, and any document prepared for distribution outside the health center. All patients in treatment with a trainee will give informed consent, which shall be documented in their charts.

SLIDING FEE ASSESSMENTS

Purpose: A Sliding Fee Schedule has been developed to meet regulations that require Federally Qualified Health Centers, such as the Family Practice and Counseling Network, to charge fees according to the patient's ability to pay.

Policy: Most insurance carriers, such as Medical Assistance and Medicare, will not pay for services that are provided to the public for free. As a Federal Grant recipient, the Network must demonstrate an effort to provide services beyond the time, scope, and amount of federal funding. Grantee funding must be matched by income generated for the delivery of services. Network health care recipients are expected to pay a share of the cost of their care.

Full charge fees are determined based on the actual cost of the services provided at the Network health centers. The standard rates for services are usual and customary. Fees are intended to be high enough to encourage persons eligible for Medicaid or other insurance coverage to obtain coverage.

Patients who are covered under an insurance plan that IS NOT accepted by the Network and therefore have access to a health care provider in their health network must pay the full fee for all services provided.

Patients who are covered under an insurance plan that IS accepted by the Network, but who have chosen another medical office or physician as their Primary Care Provider, have the option of switching to the Network as their Primary Care Provider at the time of the visit OR paying full fee for all services provided.

Procedure: Patients who are uninsured or underinsured will be charged a sliding fee according to the following procedure:

1. **The individual is required to provide proof of identification, income, and number of dependents.** Acceptable proof of identification includes a valid Driver's License or a Photo Identification Card. Acceptable proof of income includes a previous year tax return, a current pay stub, or a pension check stub. Acceptable proof of dependents includes a previous year tax return or a birth certificate. If proper documentation cannot be provided, patients are charged the full charge until proof is provided. The fee assessed to minors is determined based on the parents' or guardian's income.
2. Front desk or fiscal staff determine the percentage of the full charge of the visit for which the patient is responsible based on income level and number of household members. The percentage is determined based on published poverty guidelines. The Fee Assessment Schedule is updated annually.
3. Information on income and household members is documented in the client database system.
4. The patient is asked to pay the discounted fee upon receipt of services. However, if the patient is unable to pay at the time of visit, the patient is not denied services. The fee is charged to the patient's account and collection is attempted at future visits. Statements are also mailed to patients in an attempt to collect past due balances.

Patients whose income is below 100% of the national minimum poverty standards will be asked to pay a nominal fee at the time of the visit for all services rendered.

Exceptions: Patients who are uninsured will not be charged any fee under the following circumstances:

- The patient is receiving Family Planning services and is 17 years of age or younger.
- The patient is receiving ONLY immunizations provided by Vaccines For Children. (Fees for the visit and other services provided will be assessed, however.)
- In a serious emergency, as determined by a clinician, no patient will be refused care due to an inability to pay.

MEDICAL RECORD COMPLETION AND DOCUMENTATION

Purpose: The purpose of this policy is to assure that all patient-related information is completed and documented in the computerized or paper clinical record system.

Policy: A complete record will be kept for every patient of basic information, diagnoses, treatments recommended, and services provided. Records will be accessible and easily located, whether in paper or electronic form, and confidentiality will be carefully maintained. The person in each site with responsibility for the records will have medical records training. Records will be reviewed regularly on a random basis for completeness, quality, and legibility. Records will be properly stored and purged.

Primary Care: The Family Practice and Counseling Network utilizes an Electronic Medical Record, a computerized clinical record, for primary care. For confidentiality, it is password protected. The capability to print paper copies of records exists. A paper chart is also maintained for filing of outside reports. Paper records are stored in locked cabinets or drawers.

Behavioral Health: Paper charts are maintained for Behavioral Health patients, though computers may be used to generate documents. For policies and procedures governing the creation, maintenance, storage, organization, content, and confidentiality of Behavioral Health Charts, refer to the Mental Health, Drug and Alcohol, and CBH policy manuals located in the Behavioral Health Department.

Procedures:

Confidentiality:

All records are stored, handled and maintained in a confidential manner at all times.

- Records should never be left unattended. A screen saver protects computerized records.
- Only appropriate medical, nursing, and ancillary staff, and authorized reviewing organizations may review records.
- Written consent of the patient must be obtained if any other party or entity wants to review their records.
- Patients may review their own records at any time.

Organization:

Records must be kept in a contemporaneous manner, with entries being made consistent with regulatory and contractual requirements.

- Records should always be current for patient care.
- Written entries should be typed or legibly written in ink (black preferred).
- The provider should be identified for each note.
- The provider should sign each note.
- All progress notes, records of ancillary services, diagnostic tests, reports and letters from specialty consultants, hospital discharge summaries, and phone call records should be readily accessible.
- All entries should be dated (month, day, year).

Patient Information:

The following information should be included in an easily accessible form and location in the chart:

- Name
- Address
- Phone Number
- Marital Status
- Care-giver's information (if applicable)
- Current medications
- Visible Allergy Alerts
- Significant drug reactions
- Major or significant diseases and conditions should be documented on a "Problem List"

Maintenance of Records:

On-site files are purged annually and closed files are placed in storage. Records are maintained and preserved in accord with regulations for seven (7) years for non-prenatal records and 28 years for prenatal records.

Progress Notes:

All progress notes should indicate the following information:

- Symptoms
- Scope of examination
- Assessment (working diagnosis)
- Treatment plan
- Follow-up
- Timeframes for follow-up, indicated in days, weeks, months, or PRN (as needed)

Lab and X-Ray Tests:

Information on all diagnostic lab and x-ray tests should include:

- Name of provider who ordered the test
- Results (initialed by the provider who ordered the test)
- Follow-up action required
- Follow-up action taken

Hospitalizations:

Information on all in-patient services should include:

- Reason for admission
- Communications from specialists and other providers
- Discharge summaries
- Post-discharge action required
- Post-discharge follow-up action

Phone Contact:

Notes, phone slips, or typed computer entries to record all phone contact should be initialed and included in the record.

Appointments:

All cancellations, changes, and same-day no-shows should be included in the record.

Patient Records:

Records of children should contain the following information:

- Complete immunizations record (birth to 13 years)
- Notation of discussion of drug and alcohol use and sexual activity (over 12 years)
- Notation of discussion of tobacco use by patient (over 12 years) and caregiver (under 12 years)

Risk Management:

- Errors may be corrected by drawing a single line through the error. "White out" or markers that obscure writing should not be used to correct errors.
- Consent forms should be signed by the patient, witnessed, and included in the chart.
- Automated systems must have up-to-date anti-virus protection and must be backed up daily.
- Back-up materials must be stored off health center premises.

(*Also see RHD Policy #610—Dispute Resolution)

RIGHTS AND RESPONSIBILITIES OF PATIENTS

The Family Practice & Counseling Network Health Centers believe in the worth and dignity of all human beings.

Our Patients Have the Right to:

As our patient, you have the right to:

- Receive appointments in a timely manner.
- Be informed of all important health information and participate fully in decisions about your treatment.
- Receive care in an environment that is clean and safe.
- Receive sensitive and respectful treatment at all times.
- Speak to a Primary Care or Behavioral Health Provider after hours if you have an urgent medical problem.
- Receive confidential care in a private space.
- Express concerns to a supervisory person if you are dissatisfied with your care.
- Change health care providers.

Our Patients Have the Responsibility to:

As our patient, you have the responsibility to:

- Act in a safe manner and do not bring any firearms into the Health Center.
- Keep all scheduled appointments with the Health Center or the van service and cancel with at least one day notice.
- Treat Health Center staff with respect.
- Ask questions of the clinical staff in order to be informed of issues pertaining to your health.
- Take good care of yourself and your family . . . for you are precious.

We value you, your family, and our staff. Respectful and peaceful behavior is expected in the center at all times.

PARENTAL CONSENT FOR MINORS

Purpose: The purpose of this policy is to give a detailed explanation as to the protocol that the Family Practice and Counseling Network Health Centers uses to treat minors.

Policy: A parent or guardian is expected to be present or provide written permission to treat children under the age of 18, except in the legal situation described below. A nurse or behavioral health clinician must approve any other exceptions.

Legal Exceptions:

- A potentially life-threatening situation, where the delay of medical care could put a minor at serious risk, or where the patient is at imminent risk of harming him/herself or others.
- A person who has graduated from high school, and is married or has been pregnant, may give effective consent for medical, dental, and health services for

him/herself and the consent of no other person shall be necessary.

- Any minor may give effective consent for medical and health services to determine the presence of or treat pregnancy or venereal and other reportable diseases under the Disease Prevention and Control Law, and the consent of no other person shall be necessary.
- A minor of any age may seek drug and alcohol treatment without parental consent.
- According to state law, a minor 14 years of age or older cannot be committed involuntarily by a parent. A minor 14 years of age or older has some control of his/her mental health records and parents should not see their minor's mental health record without consent of the minor. A minor age 18 or older may seek outpatient mental health treatment independent of a parent or guardian. A minor between the ages of 14 and 18 may seek inpatient treatment without the consent of a parent. However, the consent of at least one parent or legal guardian is sought for outpatient treatment.

SERVICES TO CLIENTS WITH LIMITED ENGLISH PROFICIENCY AND HEARING IMPAIRMENTS

Purpose: The purpose of this policy is to assure that Family Practice and Counseling Network staff are able to effectively communicate with non-hearing, speech impaired, and Limited English Proficient persons to ensure their understanding of information regarding their medical conditions and treatment, their rights, and payment requirements.

Policy: It is the policy of the Family Practice and Counseling Network that no person will be denied equal access to services based solely on his/her inability to communicate aurally or verbally in the English language.

Guidelines: The non-hearing/speech impaired and Limited English Proficient patient is made aware, at the entry point for services, that he/she may request the services of an interpreter, or other appropriate communication aids, provided by the facility. A patient's request for communication assistance will be noted in his or her record. The Network ensures that the health centers have ready access to interpreter resources. The Network pays all costs incurred through the use of a contract interpreter.

Staff members are instructed that it is the **facility's obligation** to ensure effective communication with non-hearing/speech impaired and Limited English Proficient persons, not the patient's responsibility. **All staff members are instructed not to require or request that patients utilize family members, especially children, or friends as sign or foreign language interpreters. Family or friends' emotional involvement with the patient can jeopardize translation of critical medical information.** Also, family or friends may not be adequately versed in the medical terminology required for communication between patient and health professionals. Patient's own interpreters should only be used at the request of the patient. This request will be noted in the patient's medical record. Similarly, staff members are instructed not to utilize other persons awaiting services in the waiting area as interpreters. Non-hearing/speech impaired and Limited English Proficient persons, like the general public, have a right to keep information about their health status confidential.

At the time that a staff member becomes aware that a sign or foreign language interpreter is needed, an on-site management team member will be asked to approve the request. The staff member will then contact one of the resources listed below.

Interpreter Resources:

Limited English Proficiency
Interpreter Service
Nationalities Service Center
1300 Spruce Street
Philadelphia, PA 19107
215-893-8400

Non-hearing/Speech Impaired
The Communications Connection, Inc.
101 W. Airy Street
Norristown, PA 19401
Voice: 610-272-4948
TTY: 610-272-5452

Alternate Service: Deaf/Hearing Communications Center: 610-604-0425

COMPLAINTS AND GRIEVANCES

Purpose: The purpose of this policy is to outline how the Network will handle complaints and grievances from clients.

Policy: Any person or family receiving services from the Family Practice and Counseling Network has the right to be heard on grievances related to his or her treatment. It is Network policy that *IMMEDIATE* attention will be given to all grievances. Any person or family who files a grievance will be able to do so without fear of retaliation.

For the purpose of this policy, a grievance is considered to be a complaint by a person served or his/her family regarding a problem in service delivery that is *substantial and cannot be resolved in the initial contact regarding it.* Each grievance is resolved as quickly as possible and the client is informed of the resolution.

Grievances are reviewed as part of the Quality Improvement process. Any patterns or problematic cases that may result in liability for the agency will be brought to the attention of RHD through that process.

Procedure: A complaint is received from a client through an in-person contact, a telephone call, or a written communication. However the complaint is received, it will be referred to the supervisor of the staff person involved. The Responsible Supervisor will attempt to resolve the problem during an initial conversation. If that is not possible, the client will be provided with a copy of this procedure and encouraged to submit his or her grievance in writing. Anyone who needs assistance will be accommodated.

All written grievances are given to the Responsible Supervisor and the Department Director for evaluation and action as soon as possible. The Network Director is to be notified that a grievance has been filed and action is taking place. The Supervisor and Primary Care Director will attempt to resolve the grievance. The Department Director and the Network Director will then review the written grievance and a written summary of actions already taken. If the complaint has been resolved to the satisfaction of the client, the Grievance process is completed.

If dissatisfaction remains, the Network Executive Director convenes a Grievance Committee Hearing to review the grievance. The Grievance Committee consists of the Network Director and staff members appointed by the Network Director who are not involved in the grievance. The Committee will make a final decision and a response in writing. A copy of this will be shared with the individual and/or family and with any staff members involved. Any disagreement with the final decision that the individual and/or family may have will be noted in the case record and reported as such to the worker.

In the event that the decision is not satisfactory to the individual and/or family, he/she is informed that further appeals may be made by contacting RHD.

When a complaint or grievance has been resolved, it may be most appropriate to notify the person served in person or by phone of the action taken. *In all instances,* however, a written communication conveying the resolution of the complaint will be sent as well.

The Primary Care Director maintains a file of all grievances, as well as the written response regarding resolution.

Copies of all grievance documentations are sent to the Network Executive Director, and are kept on file. The Primary Care Director assures that all grievances are reviewed as part of the QI process.

CONFIDENTIALITY

Purpose: All patients have the right to confidential health care as stated in the Network mission and in accord with the provision of a safe and secure environment for patients. Network employees will have training in and will comply with the Health Information Privacy and Portability Act (HIPAA).

Policy: In the course of employment at the Network health centers, employees may have access to confidential medical and mental health information concerning Network clients. This information is obtained and recorded for the purpose of treatment. This information may only be accessed and used for the purpose of the job responsibilities of the employee. Under no circumstances will any information be disclosed by an employee about any client at the Health Centers to non-authorized personnel. All staff members will observe the right of patients to confidentiality when participating in case discussions, consultations, examinations, and treatment programs. All of these activities are to be conducted discreetly.

All Network employees will be required upon hire to read and sign a Confidentiality Statement regarding this policy.

Any violation of this policy may be considered grounds for immediate termination of employment with the Family Practice and Counseling Network. Any questions regarding this policy should be directed to the Executive Director of the Network.

• See also HIPAA requirements.

CONFLICT RESOLUTION

Purpose: The purpose of this policy is to clarify to all employees the steps they are expected to take when a conflict arises on the job.

Policy: While the Network recognizes that conflicts are a normal part of the human experience, we are committed to holding each other accountable for following a **respectful and productive** path towards the resolution of any conflict in the workplace. When conflicts are left unresolved, the entire Practice suffers the negative consequences. Refusal to participate in the resolution of a conflict is not acceptable.

When a conflict arises, the individuals involved should make every effort to meet together in a private space—away from clients/patients and other employees—to directly discuss the nature of the conflict and brainstorm ways to resolve it in a mutually satisfactory manner. When either employee feels that this communication has been unsatisfactory, they may ask for assistance from any supervisor, any management team member, or the Citizen Advocate.

If a satisfactory resolution is still not achieved, the individual may refer to the RHD Corporate Dispute Resolution procedure (Policy #610) and request a formal grievance hearing with corporate personnel.

The following are Guiding Principles established by the Network to support staff who are in conflict with one another:

1. When things get heated, ask what is really going on—get the real issue on the table.
2. When buttons get pushed, say it aloud before reacting.
3. Talk to each other with the assumption that everyone is doing the best they can.
4. Provide feedback if the tone sounds critical.

CHILD ABUSE REPORTING

Purpose: The purpose of this policy is to inform all Network employees of the requirements for reporting any suspected or alleged child abuse to the proper authorities.

Policy: In Pennsylvania, an **abused child** is defined as a child under the age of 18 who is a victim of serious non-accidental physical or mental injury, sexual abuse or exploitation, or serious physical neglect caused by the parents, a person responsible for the child's welfare, any individual residing in the same home as the child, or a parent's substitute. All Network staff must report any suspicions they have that a child is being abused or neglected, as required by law. As part of Child Protective Services' investigation of a report of suspected child abuse or neglect, Network staff may be asked for information. All staff must provide whatever assistance they can to the investigation.

Clinicians

All *clinicians* of the Family Practice and Counseling Network are mandated (by state law) to report any suspected

or alleged child abuse to the ChildLine and Abuse Registry within 24 hours by calling: 1-800-932-0313.**Mandated reporters**—as defined by Pennsylvania law—are those persons who in the course of their employment, occupation, or practice of their profession come into contact with children and must report to ChildLine when they have reason to believe, *on the basis of their medical, professional, or other training and experience*, that a child coming before them has been abused or neglected.

It is NOT the responsibility of the clinician or any other health center employee to determine the validity of suspicions or allegations. Suspicion alone is enough to warrant a call to ChildLine. Once a report is made, Child Protective Services will take responsibility for conducting an investigation and reaching a conclusion. Under no circumstances should any promise be made to keep suspicious or known information about child abuse **confidential or secret.**

Outreach and Non-Clinical Staff

All non-clinical staff members of the Network are required to notify a Network clinician *within 24 hours* if they suspect a child is being abused. Under no circumstances should any staff make a promise to keep suspicious or known information about child abuse **confidential or secret**. Only a trained professional may question a child about issues related to abuse—so DO NOT conduct your own investigation. *Suspicion alone is enough to warrant a report to a clinician and to ChildLine*.

REPORTING ALLEGED OR SUSPECTED ELDER ABUSE

Purpose: The purpose of this policy is to give employees clear information to identify possible elder abuse and to take appropriate action.

Policy: It is the policy of the Family Practice and Counseling Network that employees are mandated to report any suspected abuse of an elderly person by calling:

(215) 765-9033—Protective Services
24 hours per day—7 days per week

All clinicians of the Network must report any suspected or alleged elder abuse as soon as possible. Non-clinical staff are required to notify a Network clinician *within 24 hours* if they suspect an older patient is being abused.

The Pennsylvania Older Adults Protective Services Act provides the following terms and definitions:

- **Abuse: The occurrence of one or more of the following acts:**

  - The infliction of injury, unreasonable confinement, intimidation, or punishment with resulting physical harm, pain, or mental anguish.
  - The willful deprivation by a caretaker of goods or services which are necessary to maintain physical or mental health.
  - Sexual harassment, rape, or abuse, as defined in the Protection Form Abuse Act (35 P.S. 10181-10190).

No older adult will be found to be abused solely on the grounds of environmental factors which are beyond the control of the older adult or the caretaker, such as inadequate housing, furnishing, income, clothing, or medical care.

- **Caretaker:** An individual or institution that has assumed the responsibility for the provision of care needed to maintain the physical or mental health of an older adult. This responsibility may arise voluntarily, by contract, by receipt of payment for care, as a result of family relationship, or by order of a court of competent jurisdiction. It is not the intent of the Act to impose responsibility on an individual if the responsibility would not otherwise exist in law.
- **Older Adult:** An individual within the jurisdiction of this Commonwealth who is 60 years of age or older.
- **Older Adult in Need of Protective Services:** An incapacitated older adult who is unable to perform or obtain services that are necessary to maintain physical or mental health, for which there is no responsible caretaker and who is at imminent risk of danger to his/her person or property.

CULTURAL COMPETENCE

Purpose: Because all of the individuals and families who come to the Family Practice and Counseling Network for services come with cultural influences from their backgrounds, the staff at the Network must strive to be culturally competent in the performance of their duties and to recognize, respect, and respond to the unique, culturally-defined needs of the consumers. The Network management and staff strive to incorporate cultural knowledge into policy-making and practice.

Policy: The Network finds the following principles to be important to the provision of culturally competent services.

- Cultural competence involves working in conjunction with natural, informal support, and helping networks within the community.
- Cultural competence extends the concept of self-determination to the community.
- Individuals and families may make different choices based on cultural forces.
- Inherent in cross-cultural interactions are dynamics that will be acknowledged and accepted.
- A staffing pattern that reflects the make-up of the population helps ensure the delivery of effective services.
- Culturally competent services incorporate the concept of equal and nondiscriminatory services, but include the concept of services that are responsive to the population served.

Cultural competence is the ability to deal with an individual or family in a way that they feel comfortable that their feelings and actions will be understood. Cultural competence creates an environment in which people of different cultures can understand one another and can communicate across cultures, not so much by words, as by a respect and knowledge of how culture influences such things as child rearing, sense of time, and priorities of living. Cultural competence assumes knowledge of how economic circumstances affect what people will do under certain conditions and provides meaning to what some may think of as unreasonable behavior.

Procedures: The Network will provide training regarding cultural competence issues to give staff the tools and the opportunity to clarify any questions or issues they may have. There will be training for new staff around the cultures most often served. The goal of the training will be to give staff members a greater understanding of the motivations and priorities of different cultures and help them to give nurturing and helpful support to individuals, children, and families of different cultures. Training will include:

- Cultural and ethnic differences and responsive strategies most effective with the groups served by the agency;
- Interventions that address cultural and socioeconomic class factors in service delivery;
- The role cultural identity plays in motivating human behavior;
- Differences in norms and values;
- Personal and institutionalized bias or discrimination; and

- The application of cultural variables in differential diagnosis/assessment and in designing responsive interventions.

CODE BLUE

Purpose: The purpose of this procedure is to communicate to staff the proper and rapid response to any life-threatening situation that may occur at a Network health center.

Policy: The Family Practice and Counseling Network has determined the use of the term "CODE BLUE" to alert all center staff that their **immediate presence is required** at a designated location. A situation requiring the announcement of a CODE BLUE exists when there is a perception on the part of staff that there is imminent threat of death.

Some examples are:

- A suicide attempt has occurred or is about to occur.
- There is a cardiac arrest occurring or about to occur.
- There is a respiratory arrest occurring or about to occur.
- There is a threat of violence.

Procedure:

1. A CODE BLUE may be called by anyone who believes that any of the above is occurring or about to occur. Using the telephone paging system, the caller will announce "CODE BLUE" **and specify the exact location**. All staff must report to that location immediately and remain there until dismissed by a Crisis Team member or leading clinician.
2. Although any individual may call a CODE BLUE, the management of the situation must be turned over to the clinician present who is most senior with the Network as soon as possible.
3. The senior clinician will assume the leadership of the situation and **will give orders to staff as to specific tasks.**
4. All staff are expected to follow all orders given and continue to be present until dismissed by the leading clinician. This is NOT the time to question authority. Debriefing and questioning of authority may occur after a CODE BLUE has ceased. Failure to carry out an order exactly as directed during a CODE BLUE may result in immediate termination of employment.
5. A CODE BLUE ceases only when the leading clinician calls it off.
6. Any CODE BLUE situation must be reported as soon as possible to the Executive Director of the Network and must be documented on an Incident Reporting Form.

CRISIS MANAGEMENT

Purpose: The purpose of this policy is to define a crisis and outline the specific action to be taken in the event of a crisis.

Policy: The health center staff will respond to a crisis in a brisk and systematic manner in order to support those who are or may be affected by a crisis.

What Is a Crisis?

A crisis is an unanticipated event that is having or has the potential of having a profound physical or emotional impact on one or more members of the health center staff, health center clients, the community, or the physical space of the health center. A crisis may occur as the result of an unexpected serious injury, illness, death, or destruction to property.

What Is the Crisis Team?

Members of the Senior Management Team, as well as the leading clinician during a "CODE BLUE," constitute the Crisis Team.

What Is the Response to a Crisis?

When a crisis occurs, it is the responsibility of any staff member present to act swiftly to alleviate the immediate affects of the crisis. This may be to call 911, call a "CODE BLUE," call on a member of the Crisis Team for help, or administer CPR. It is the responsibility of the staff member who took action to notify the Network Director or another member of the Crisis Team (described above) about the crisis as soon as possible.

What Is the Responsibility of the Crisis Team?

The Crisis Team will assume the following responsibilities:

- Promptly communicate to each member of the Team
- Determine needs/tasks
- Assign individuals to accomplish tasks

Tasks may include, but are not limited to, the following: provision of emotional support to individual staff or community members, communication to tenant council and/or community or other appropriate people, obtaining information (as in the case of communicable disease), arranging emergency transport as needed, and documenting the incident, where appropriate.

HOSPITALIZATION

Purpose: The purpose of this policy is to ensure that all patients requiring emergency attention are expeditiously referred to the nearest Emergency Room for the specialized care needed and that continuity of care is maintained.

Policy: Network health center patients requiring emergency evaluation for hospital admission will be referred to the nearest emergency room. Whenever possible, the health center will provide transportation or will assure safe transportation via 911 or a family member. Emergency Room staff will be called ahead of time to facilitate care for the patient. If the patient is admitted to the hospital, the house staff or the Network's contracting physician may care for them. If possible, the Nurse Practitioner or Registered Nurse from the health center will round on the patient and, if not, will maintain contact with the patient and or the providers caring for him/her and will obtain a discharge summary in order to provide a continuity of care.

In some instances, the patient may be directly admitted and followed by one of the center's consulting physicians. At a minimum, the health center clinician will maintain close contact with the patient during hospitalization.

INCIDENT REPORTING POLICY

Purpose: Incident reporting is an important means of communicating events that have actual or potential consequences on the health, safety, or well being of our customers, health centers, or Network as a whole. Incident reporting is also required by some funders and regulators.

Recording of significant events allows important issues to be revealed, investigated and resolved in a systematic way. It also provides structured opportunities for change and improvements made possible through knowledge gained. Reporting should therefore be viewed as a positive and helpful action, and not as punitive or negative.

The purpose of this policy is to define classes of reportable incidents, and procedures to be utilized by all staff to report unusual or adverse events involving staff, patients,

visitors, and anyone else associated with the operations or property of the health centers.

Policy: It is the policy of FPCN that all incidents involving health center staff or user be documented, reported and investigated utilizing the FPCN incident reporting procedure outlined in this policy. Incidents are reviewed a minimum of quarterly as part of the FPCN Quality Improvement process.

Scope: This policy pertains to all sites.

Definitions:

Incident—any event that causes actual or potential harm, physical or emotional, to a health center user or employee and is inconsistent with the normal or expected operations of the health center.

Examples include, but not limited to the following:

- Falls
- Needle sticks or exposure to blood borne pathogens
- Medication errors
- Injury while performing normal work duties
- Injury resulting from equipment malfunction
- A threat or assault causing physical harm or psychological distress
- Emergencies requiring the calling of 9-1-1 for Police, Ambulance, or Fire
- Theft or property damage
- Customer complaints
- Child abuse, neglect, sexual abuse
- Other incidents or events noted on Philadelphia Behavioral Health System "Significant Incident Report" form found in the CBH policy and procedure manual.

Customer—employees, patients, visitors, or vendors.

Procedure:

1. *Reporting incidents*
   - Incidents are reported to a supervisor immediately, or, if non-urgent in nature, no later than 24 hours from the occurrence. *Incidents involving CBH or other county funded Mental Health clients must also be reported to CBH and OMH within 24 hours.*
   - The person(s) most directly involved in the event, or the person or persons that observed or discovered the event are responsible for filing the report in a timely manner.
   - If necessary, the supervisor will assist in the completion of the form.

2. *Documentation*

- The incident is documented on the Incident Reporting Form (Attachment A) and/or the CBH "Significant Incident Report"—if deemed necessary by Behavioral Health Department personnel (Attachment C).
- The information and completed form are treated in a confidential manner and never photocopied or duplicated.
- The report is to be completed legibly and objectively with only the facts.
- Personal comments and opinions are not included on the form.
- Employees will refrain from discussing any event with persons not directly involved and observe rules associated with patient/employee confidentiality.
- Forms are located at the front desk, in the Network Policy Manual, CQI manual, and the CBH Manual. All supervisors keep blank forms that are available upon request.

3. *Submitting, follow-up, and disposition of Incident Reports*

- All incidents are reported to the immediate supervisor. If the immediate supervisor is unavailable, the next level of management is notified.
- The Departmental Director and Network Executive Director are notified within 24 hrs.
- The Department Director and/or designated supervisor, receive all Incident Report forms generated by his or her staff or that pertains to his or her department operations.
- Follow-up investigation is conducted by the Department Director and/or designated supervisor *within 72 hours of receipt of the form.* Documentation of investigation, follow up, and action(s) taken are completed on the Incident Report Follow-up form (Attachment B).
- The Performance Improvement Committee Chair and Network Executive Director are forwarded the completed Incident Report and Follow-up Form.
- Further follow-up or investigation is conducted by the Performance Improvement Committee Chair, or Network Executive Director, if indicated.
- Significant findings, conclusions, actions and recommendations will be communicated to RHD and the Board if indicated. This is the responsibility of the Network Executive Director or designee through established procedures.
- Incident reports are maintained by the Performance Improvement Committee Chair and data reports generated a minimum of quarterly, and reported out to the Senior Leadership team and Performance Improvement Committee.

SENIOR MANAGEMENT TEAM GUIDELINES FOR OPERATION

Purpose: The purpose of this policy is to describe the make-up of the Family Practice and Counseling Network Senior Management Team, hereafter referred to as the Management Team, and to outline how the members of that team operate with regard to one another, the Network health centers, the Network Advisory Board, and RHD. It also serves as information to all staff on issues pertaining to governance of the health centers.

Policy:

I. **Who comprises the Management Team?**
   The Management Team consists of the Executive Director, Primary Care Director, Behavioral Health Director, Business Director, Fiscal Director, Eleventh Street Director, and Administrative Director. It is possible that other department directors could be added to this team depending on the scope of services, size, and make-up of staff in their department. All major departments must be represented on the Management Team.

II. **What is the frequency of meetings for the Management Team?**
   The Management Team meets formally at least twice a month for approximately 3 hours each meeting. The entire team or members of the team will meet more often as needed.

III. **What are the overall responsibilities of the Management Team?**
   The Management Team is responsible for the governance and management of the operations of the Network health centers, including the formation and enforcement of policies and procedures; the hiring, disciplining, and termination of staff; the allocation of resources; and the creation, direction, and evaluation of the strategic plan.

IV. **How does the Management Team make decisions?**
   The Network embraces RHD values: multilevel thinking, empowerment of groups, and decentraliza-

tion of authority. These values drive the health center Management Team operations. Input of all staff or groups is frequently sought as a matter of course in multiple aspects of Network operations, programmatic design, and personnel policy.

Decisions may be made in one of several ways: consensus of the Management Team; a department director in collaboration with other team members; the Network Executive Director or department director alone; some—but not all—Management Team members; or in conjunction with the Network Advisory Board or RHD. The Network Executive Director is the point person who is accountable to RHD and the Network Advisory Board and, for this reason, may at times make sole decisions that are felt to be in the best interest of the Network. These decisions can be challenged.

A. **Consensus**—It is understood that not all decisions can be made by consensus; however, when all members of the Management Team can get behind a major action plan, it has a positive impact on the entire organization. Therefore, attempts are made to attain consensus whenever possible on: major policy or procedure that impacts consumers, significant allocation of resources such as money or space, program cuts or expansion, adding a new position, and other issues having a major impact on overall operating costs and affecting the financial health of the Network.

B. **Department Director in collaboration with Executive Director and/or other members of the team**—Termination or major discipline of a member of a director's department and significant departmental policy changes affecting clinical care or departmental operations are decisions made largely by department directors. In accord with RHD policy, termination of an employee must include concurrence by at least one other person of equal or higher authority. However, the Network Executive Director (Eleventh St. Director for Drexel employees) must support the decision to terminate or significantly discipline an employee or to change significant departmental policy.

C. **Department Director alone**—Decisions regarding usual day-to-day operations that do not have substantial impact on resources or involve major policy change affecting staff or patients are made by department directors alone.

D. **RHD involvement**—RHD involvement occurs in the creation and monitoring of the Network budget and when an issue presents a possible legal action against the Network or RHD, when there is intent to terminate an employee, and when there is a significant change in scope or location of services. RHD may be brought into the process at the discretion of the Network Executive Director when a significant ethical or legal conundrum exists. Other members of the Management Team may likewise request the involvement of RHD in conjunction with the Director, unless there is significant conflict or questioning of the behavior of the Director on the part of another management team member. In that case, the Management Team member may go to RHD without first collaborating with the Network Executive Director. For parallel issues at Eleventh Street, Drexel protocol is followed.

E. **Health Center Advisory Board**—In accord with the Memorandum of Understanding, a legal agreement that was initially made between Abbottsford Homes Tenant Management Corporation and RHD and continues to dictate the relationship between the Network Advisory Board and RHD, the Advisory Board will be involved in the following decisions:

1. Those that involve significant alterations of the physical space belonging to the Philadelphia Housing Authority, such as major renovations, expansion to new buildings or spaces, and changes to the exterior appearance of a building;

2. Major policy changes;

3. Expenditures or other obligations that, when added to other expenditures for the fiscal year, exceed the Network budget or any category specified in the budget by 15% of the approved annual budget;

4. The Network Executive Director or another Management Team member will seek the input of resident leaders who serve on the Network Advisory Board regarding the hiring of a housing development resident as a health center staff member.

V. **What is the protocol for Challenging Decisions that are made?**

There must be freedom among the Management Team members to request clarification and challenge decisions made by the Network Executive Director or any other member of the Management Team. In challenging a decision, Management Team members should first attempt to resolve issues among themselves before involving a higher authority such as RHD. Likewise, any staff member must be empowered to request clarification or challenge decisions made by any member of the Management Team, but they too are encouraged to first go to their own supervisor prior to taking their concerns to a higher authority. This does not discount any staff person's right to take an issue to any person they choose. The issue of challenging decisions is discussed in more detail in the RHD Personnel Policies (see Values section).

VI. **Management Team Committees**

The Management Team may have committees consisting of smaller numbers of people who address, research, and/or make final decisions on certain issues. This is not intended to undermine the entire team, but rather to streamline processes and provide for a smaller body to make final decisions on key issues. One such committee is the Fiscal Committee. The role of this committee is to make final decisions on new sites, existing site expansion, new hires, budget approval, grant applications, salaries and compensation, and days of operation. Other standing or ad hoc committees may develop as needed. The Executive Director must approve of the formation and function of Management Team committees.

RECRUITMENT AND RETENTION OF STAFF

Purpose: The purpose of this policy is to inform employees of the ways in which the Network tries to attract new personnel and successfully retain them.

Policy:

Recruitment of Staff

Family Practice and Counseling is committed to giving priority to qualified candidates for employment who are also residents of the housing communities we serve. Tenant leaders are consulted regarding the hiring of residents.

Recruitment procedures include posting the position with the Unemployment office; distributing flyers door-to-door in the community; placing additional flyers in strategic communal areas; placing advertisements in newspapers, journals, and professional e-mail list services; and word of mouth. Advertisements and postings reflect that we are an Equal Opportunity Employer. Potential candidates must demonstrate a commitment and desire to work in a health care setting that provides health care to an underserved population. They must have references that indicate personal character traits and competence compatible with the job requirements. A credentialing committee must approve clinical staff.

Retention of Staff

The Family Practice and Counseling Network makes every effort to retain quality staff and to offer staff the opportunity to advance within the Network. When staff members leave the organization, a formal exit interview is held to help the Network determine why people are leaving and what suggestions those people can make or what their experiences might suggest to improve retention. Other strategies to assure the lowest turnover rate possible are:

Orientation—All staff are oriented to the health centers' policies and procedures and receive a copy of the manual. They are also oriented to the clinical practice guideline manual, laboratory manual, and behavioral health procedures as indicated by their health center position. An orientation checklist is utilized to record observations and to assure all defined items are addressed and completed satisfactorily.

Participation in Network Activities—Clinical staff attend regular meetings that include case conferences and problem solving and support sessions. Staff are asked to serve on committees such as CQI, national committees for quality improvement in chronic illness and wellness care, patient flow committees, and other ad hoc or problem-solving forums. All staff meetings call for staff participation in problem identification and resolution, creation of policies, improved communication, and the celebration of good works.

Continuing Education/Professional Development—Clinical staff are encouraged to seek additional skills training and expected to earn the CEUs required for their positions. They are provided paid time and reimbursement for conference expenses as the budget allows. They are expected to share their education with other clinical staff. Clinicians have the opportunity to teach and are provided the opportunity to be adjunct faculty at local colleges/universities and receive the accompanying benefits afforded this position. Clinicians also have the opportunity to represent the health centers by presenting at conferences, participating in research and or program evaluation, and providing relevant testimonies on behalf of health issues and policy. All staff receive in-service presentations and continuing education pertinent to their positions. All RHD employees are eligible to attend a variety of professional and personal courses offered through the RHD Miniversity, which are free of charge to employees.

Exit Interviews—The Network conducts an exit interview with all personnel who leave voluntarily. This interview enables staff to address administrative issues related to the transition, as well as to receive feedback on the organization's strengths and weaknesses.

PROFESSIONAL LIABILITY

Purpose: The purpose of this policy is to clarify the requirements for malpractice insurance coverage.

Policy: The Network requires that all clinicians be covered by malpractice insurance. All health center employees **who are on the RHD payroll** are deemed under the Federal Tort Claim Act (FTCA) and are therefore covered (at no cost to the employee) by this federal insurance for any malpractice claims brought against them.

Consultants are NOT always considered deemed—and therefore are NOT covered under this Act. The Network will specify as part of the contract whether a consultant is covered, depending on FTCA regulations, and will determine on a case-by-case basis whether the Network will pay for any part or all of the consultant's malpractice insurance premium.

CREDENTIALING OF PRIMARY CARE NURSE PRACTITIONERS/PHYSICIANS/DENTISTS

Policy: It is the policy of the Family Practice & Counseling Network that all licensed or certified health care practitioners are assessed through a specific and formal process, with the ultimate goal being the safe and competent care of all health center patients.

Purpose:

1. To assure the patients of Family Practice & Counseling Network hereinafter referred to as FPCN, are receiving care from individuals who reflect the highest levels of qualifications and competencies in their respective professional disciplines.
2. Meet Federal standards and policy requirements (see Appendix I).

Scope: This policy applies to all individuals permitted, by law, to provide patient care services with or without direct supervision, within the scope of their licenses and individually granted clinical privileges.

Definition: Credentialing is the process of obtaining, verifying and assessing the qualifications of a health care practitioner to provide patient care services in our organization. Clinicians are credentialed to ensure the safety of patients and to comply with regulatory requirements.

Responsibility: FPCN will appoint and re-appoint appropriately licensed and qualified individuals to the dental/primary care staff and will grant such individuals specific clinical privileges. Such appointments and reappointments will be made upon the recommendation(s) of the Primary Care Director (PCD), or Dental Director. The gathering of the necessary documentation is the responsibility of the Human Resources Officer. The assessing of the necessary documentation is the responsibility of the PCD, or Dental Director.

The FPCN will be responsible for maintaining appropriate and secure files containing all relevant information related to the credentialing and/or privileging of the nursing/medical/dental staff.

Specific Procedures:

CREDENTIALING—The decision to appoint or re-appoint an individual to the PC/Dental staff will be governed by the presence of verified documentation of the following core criteria:

1. **Current Licensure**—is verified at the time of employment by viewing the applicant's original (not a copy) current license or registration.
2. **Relevant Training and Experience**—FPCN will verify relevant training and experience from the primary source(s).
3. **Background Checks**—A statement signed by the practitioner declaring that the he/she has never been convicted of a felony, is not under investigation for suspected commission of a felony, is not under investigation by the board of nursing, medicine or dentistry for a licensing offense, and has not been

suspended from Medicaid or Medicare provider status. Other verifications include child abuse clearance and criminal background check and a statement of the practitioner's malpractice history. The National Practitioner Data Bank (NPDB) keeps records of all damage awards for medical malpractice paid by a practitioner. A practitioner can get his or her own report by requesting a form from the NPDB. Hospitals can subscribe to the service. Actions by state boards of nursing are not required to be reported by NPs, but reporting is required for MDs and DDSs.

4. **State Board Requirements**—The practice agreement under which the practitioner is practicing, if applicable.

    Prescribing authority. Providers need to obtain Drug Enforcement Administration (DEA) numbers (410-962-7580) and state Controlled Dangerous Substance (CDS) numbers. Nurse Practitioners must obtain prescription privileges according to the regulations outlined by the Pa. State Board of Nursing.

5. **Verifications**—A copy of two professional references, including name, address, telephone number, title, nature of professional association with employee, and recommendation as to clinical competence and ability to work with a team.

    This includes letters from professional schools (for example, nursing/dental/or medical). Board certification in medical specialties is confirmed by the listing in the official ABMS Directory of Board Certified Medical Specialists. Board certification in dental specialties is supported by appropriate documentation. A copy of the signed job description and current curriculum vitae/resume is kept on file.

FORMS: See appendix II and III

Annual Review—Each year, clinicians will have a performance evaluation regarding adherence to Network Policy and clinical practice standards, as well as:

- Verification that annual requirements for CEUs have been met.
- Query of the National Data Bank for primary care providers and physicians.
- Documentation and verification of current licenses, certifications, and registrations, if applicable.
- Documentation of active Malpractice coverage, either through the Federal Tort Claim Act or other insurance entity, according to the requirements of funders or other regulating bodies.

- Child abuse clearance and criminal background checks as required by regulations.

Appendix I—Family Practice & Counseling application for nurse practitioner/medical/dental staff appointment

Appendix II—Family Practice & Counseling Network Clinical Staff Credential/Re Credentialing* Documents Required for Provider/Employee File

APPENDIX I

FAMILY PRACTICE & COUNSELING APPLICATION FOR NURSE PRACTITIONER/MEDICAL/DENTAL STAFF APPOINTMENT

GENERAL INSTRUCTIONS:

1. If more space is needed, attach additional sheets and make reference to the questions being answered.
2. If you have not previously submitted copies of the following documents, please attach them to this application:
   a. Current License(s) to practice as a nurse practitioner, dentistry, or medicine;
   b. Narcotics (DEA) registration certificate;
   c. Professional liability insurance policy and certificate of current coverage from insurance carrier
   d. Evidence of board status (if applicable); and
   e. A curriculum vitae
   f. Physician collaborating agreement

I. PERSONAL IDENTIFICATION DATA

Name (Last)   (First)   (MI)

Date: _____

Office Address: _____

Telephone: _____

Home Address: _____

Telephone: _____

Birthdate: _____

Birthplace: _____

Medicare Provider #: _____

UPIN #: _____

Medicaid Provider #: _____

Social Security #: _____

II. PROFESSIONAL DATA

A. General Information:
   1. Clinical Specialty/Subspecialty:

   _____

   2. Other interests in practice, research, etc.:

   _____

   3. Name others with whom you are associated in practice and the nature of the association.

   _____

   _____

B. Practice Information
   Please answer each of the following questions in full. If the answer to any questions is "yes," please provide full explanation of the details on a separate sheet, and attach.

   1. Have any disciplinary actions been initiated or are any pending against you by any state licensure board?
      Yes   No

   2. Has your license to practice in any state ever been denied, limited, suspended or revoked?
      Yes   No

   3. Have you ever been suspended, sanctioned or otherwise restricted from participating in any private, federal or state health insurance program (for example, Medicare, Medicaid)?
      Yes   No

   4. Have you ever been the subject of an investigation by any private, federal or state agency concerning your participation in any private, federal or state health insurance program?
      Yes   No

   5. Has your narcotics registration certificate ever been investigated, limited, suspended or revoked?
      Yes   No

   6. Is your narcotics registration certificate currently being investigated or challenged?
      Yes   No

   7. Have you ever been named as a defendant in any type of criminal proceeding?
      Yes   No

III. EDUCATIONAL DATA

A. Schools Degree Date of Graduation

_____
Undergraduate College or University

_____
Complete Address

_____
Nursing/Medical/Dental/Podiatric College

_____
Complete Address

_____
Other Professional Training

_____
Complete Address

B. Internships/Dates

_____

| Institution | Type of Internship |

_____

| From | To | Rotating |

_____

| Name | Special |

_____
Complete Address

Other: (If more than one internship was begun or completed, please supply the same information on a separate sheet and attach.)

C. Residencies

_____

| Department | Type of | Dates |

_____

| Institution Chairperson | Residency | From | To |

_____
Name

_____
Complete Address

_____
Name

_____
Complete Address

(If more than two residencies were begun or completed, please supply the same information on a separate sheet and attach.)

D. Fellowships

_____

| Department | Type of | Dates |

_____

| Institution Chairperson | Fellowship | From | To |

Name

Complete Address

Name

Complete Address

(If more than two fellowships were begun or completed, please supply the same information on a separate sheet and attach.)

E. Teaching Appointments

Department   Type of   Dates

Institution Chairperson   Appointment   From

Name

Complete Address

(If more than one teaching appointment was begun or completed. please supply the same information on a separate sheet and attach.)

F. Post-Graduate and Continuing Education Course

(During Past Three Years) Dates

Name and Address of Institution   From

(If more space is needed, please attach separate sheet.)

IV. INSTITUTIONAL AFFILIATIONS

A. List in chronological order all institutional affiliations since completion of post-graduate education. Complete addresses must be included. If more space is needed, attach additional sheet.

Department Dates

Institution

Address

Department   From   To

Chairperson

B. Has your employment, medical staff appointment or clinical privileges ever been voluntarily or involuntarily relinquished, suspended, diminished, revoked, refused, limited or not renewed at any hospital or other health care facility?

Yes   No

C. Have you ever withdrawn your application for appointment, reappointment and clinical privileges or resigned from the medical staff before a hospital's or health care facility's governing board made a decision?

Yes   No

D. Have you ever been the subject of disciplinary proceedings at any hospital or health care facility?

Yes   No

E. Has any health care entity ever reported any malpractice payment made for your benefit, any licensure action or any adverse disciplinary action concerning you to the National Practitioner Data Bank?

Yes   No

If the answer to B, C, ,D or E is yes, please provide a full explanation of the details on a separate sheet and attach.

VI. PROFESSIONAL LIABILITY DATA

A. Insurance

1. Identify your professional liability carrier by name, address, policy number, limits of liability, expiration date:

2. Has your professional liability insurance coverage ever been terminated by action of the insurance company?

Yes   No

3. Have you ever been denied professional liability insurance coverage?

Yes   No

4. If the answer to question 1 or 2 above is yes, state when, by what company, and why:

5. Has your present professional liability insurance carrier excluded any specific procedures from your coverage?

Yes   No

6. If the answer to question 5 above is yes, list the procedures that have been excluded and provide a full explanation on a separate sheet, including the name of the carrier, the date and specific information concerning any limitation.

B. Malpractice Claims and Legal Actions

1. During the past five (5) years have you been informed of any professional liability claims (not yet suits) being made against you?

   Yes   No

2. Have any professional liability suits ever been filed against you?

   Yes   No

3. Have any professional liability suits been filed against you, which are presently pending?

   Yes   No

4. Have any verdicts, judgments or settlements been made in any professional liability case in which you have been involved?

   Yes   No

   If the answer to any of the above questions is yes, please provide a full explanation of the details on a separate sheet, and attach. If litigation was involved, the explanation must include the name of the court in which any suit was filed, the parties, caption and docket number of the case, and the name and address of the attorney defending you. Also furnish a description of the claim made against you and the outcome of the litigation. If no litigation was involved, identify the claimant and his/her attorney. Describe the claim, when it arose, what the final disposition was and the name and address of the attorney defending you.

VIII. MISCELLANEOUS

A. References

List at least two professional references and one character reference, and as many more as you like, not including relatives, current partners or associates in practice. Provide current, complete addresses. References will be evaluated according to the extent of their direct clinical observation of your work, your judgment, your ethical character, your ability to work with others and their other knowledge of you.

1. Name: _____
   Telephone: _____
   Address: _____

2. Name: _____
   Telephone: _____
   Address: _____

3. Name: _____
   Telephone: _____
   Address: _____

APPENDIX II

Family Practice & Counseling Network Clinical Staff Credential/ Re-Credentialing* Documents Required for Provider/Employee File

DOCUMENTS IN CLINICAL STAFF FILES	YES	NO
1) Professional School Diploma		
2) Certificate of Residency Training (As Applicable)		
3) Board Certification (As Applicable)		
4) Immunization Status (At Lease Hepatitis B Vaccine)		
5) PPD Status		
6) Current License to Practice		
7) DEA Registration		
8) Reference Letters (Professional & Personal—Minimum 3)		
9) Life Support Training (BLS, ACLS, ATLS, As Appropriate)		
10) Documentation of Continuing Professional Education		
11) Annual Performance Evaluation**		
12) Proof of Malpractice Insurance or FTCA		
13) National Practitioner Data Bank Inquiries**		
14) Current Employment Contract or Position Description**		
15) Collaborating Physician Agreement		

16) Any History of Professional Liability Claims/Settlements
17) Information From Relevant Organizations About Sanctions or Limitations on Licensure, or Previous Sanctions by Medicare/Medicaid (HCFA website).
18) Signed Attestation by Applicant For The Correctness and Completeness of the Application and Re-credentialing* Form
19) Statement Regarding Physical or Mental Impairments With or Without Accommodations
20) Statement Regarding Lack of Present Illegal Drug Use
21) Statement Regarding History of Loss of License or Felony Convictions
22) Statement Regarding History of Loss or Limitation of Privileges or Disciplinary Action(s)

NOTE: New and first-time Clinical Staff/Providers must have all of the above-required documents. Providers that these documents pertain to include physician, dentist, and nurse practitioner. *Re-credentialing of Clinical Staff/Providers must occur ever two years. **Documents required must be given by the Health Care Center of the Clinical Staff/Prov

PRODUCTIVITY STANDARDS

Purpose: The purpose of this policy is to set productivity standards for all clinicians that will ensure ongoing fiscal viability of the Network and maintain quality care.

Policy: Staff clinicians are expected to meet productivity standards set forth by their clinical supervisor/Department Director. Standards are reviewed annually by the Department Directors and set in consultation with the Manage-

ment Team and with the approval of the Executive Management Team and the Executive Director. Meeting productivity is a component of clinicians' performance evaluations.

EMPLOYEE PERFORMANCE EVALUATIONS

Purpose: Performance evaluations are provided at specific intervals in order to provide the following to all employees:

1. A formal means of clarifying expectations, goals, and standards.
2. An opportunity for two-way communication between supervisor and employee when presenting the evaluation of an employee's performance.
3. Data needed to make decisions regarding salary adjustments, promotions, and disciplinary actions.

Policy: The Family Practice and Counseling Network is committed to providing meaningful supervision to all employees. Providing ongoing feedback and maintaining open communication between supervisor and supervisee is crucial to successful job performance. It is in the best interest of the Network—and the people served—to ensure the individual success and personal/professional growth of all employees.

All newly hired employees will receive a formal evaluation at the end of their 90-day probation period and annually from the date of hire. Employees may be evaluated at additional times as deemed necessary by the supervisor, and ongoing, informal feedback is always encouraged and supported. All formal evaluations are presented to employees in person with time set aside for reviewing the evaluation together. All evaluations are criteria-based and allow for both positive and critical observations. Evaluations should be signed by the supervisor. Employees *must* sign their written evaluations in order to verify that the information was presented to the employee. Signing does NOT imply agreement with the supervisor's evaluation and each employee has the opportunity to document their own comments about the evaluation, as well as requesting a formal grievance hearing, if desired.

APPENDIX J

Sample Physician Collaborative Agreement

This Physician Collaborative Agreement ("Agreement") sets forth the material terms relating to the collaboration and directions services provided by Dr. _____ employed by _____ Community Health (CH) to the Certified Registered Nurse Practitioners ("CRNPs") at Health Centers, located at _____.

The Health Centers are located within public housing communities in _____. Their goal is to provide primary care, health education, and other supportive programs that will enable the health centers' users to obtain an optimal state of health. The primary care and the vast majority of the other services at the Health Centers are provided by the CRNPs in accordance with state and federal law. The services provided by the CRNPs include acts of medical diagnosis, prescription of medical therapeutics, and corrective measures, all of which are performed in collaboration with physicians licensed in Pennsylvania.

The purpose of this Agreement is to assist the Centers and CH in serving the needs of patients who are seen at the Centers and, where appropriate, to facilitate appropriate referral and transfer of these patients. It is also the purpose of this Agreement to enable the CRNPs at the Centers to practice to the fullest extent permitted under state and federal law and to facilitate reimbursement for the services provided at the Centers, including reimbursement from the Medicare and Medicaid programs. Except as set forth herein, neither CH nor its physicians assume any responsibility for the overall care of the Centers' patients by virtue of this Agreement.

1. **Term:** This agreement will be effective on September 1, 1998, for a term of six (6) months and will automatically be renewed thereafter for successive one (1) year terms unless terminated by either party upon sixty (60) days prior written notice. The effect of such notice will be to terminate all obligations of this Agreement as of midnight on the 60th day after written notice of termination is received, except the parties' obligation under paragraph 6, below.

2. **Services Provided by CH:** CH will make physician(s) available to the CRNPs at the Centers for consultation relating to the CRNPs' activities at the Centers and to assist the Centers on meeting requirements of state and federal law. These physician(s) will be duly licensed in the Commonwealth of Pennsylvania and will:

    a. Make themselves available during the Centers' regularly scheduled operating hours, as reasonably required for the care of the Centers' patients, through direct communications or by radio, telephone, or telecommunications.

    b. Develop with the CRNPs at the Centers a predetermined plan for emergency services.

    c. Make themselves available on a regularly scheduled basis for:

        1. Referrals.
        2. Reviewing the standards of medical practice incorporating consultation and chart review.
        3. Establishing and updating standing orders, drug and other medical protocols within the practice setting.
        4. Periodic updating in medical diagnosis and therapeutics.
        5. Cosigning records when necessary to document accountability by both parties.
        6. Providing other services necessary to meet Medicare and/or Medicaid requirements.

    The physician(s) agree to schedule regular hours at the centers to be present in order to carry out these functions in the case of adult medicine services, at least once every six (6) weeks.

d. CH will ensure that the physician(s) providing services under this Agreement are appropriately licensed and qualified to practice as physicians in accordance with the laws and regulations of the Commonwealth of Pennsylvania, including ongoing recertification, and shall provide evidence thereof to the Centers upon request.

3. **Responsibilities of the Centers:**

a. CH and the Centers have adopted protocols and standards to be followed by the CRNPs in the performance of services at the Centers. The Centers and CH are in accordance with the protocols and standards developed by the Community Health Network ("CHN"), Healthy People 2000 and the Clinical Regional Advisory Network ("CRAN"). In adopting these protocols and standards, CH and the Centers agree that CRNPs must be prepared by education and experience to determine when consultation or referral with other health professionals is necessary in the primary care setting. Consultation may consist of telephone contact with the collaborating physician, or site discussion, chart review, or referral for physician examination of patient.

b. If the CRNPs at the Centers determine that a patient needs emergency or urgent care, during regular business hours or after hours, the patient will be referred to the emergency room of a hospital that is appropriate in light of the needs and wishes of the patient. The Centers assume responsibility for facilitating safe transportation of the patient when urgent or emergent services are necessary.

c. The CRNPs are responsible for maintaining the clinical record to at least community standards and for facilitating each patient obtaining necessary screenings and immunizations. A CRNP is available for telephone consultation twenty-four (24) hours per day, seven (7) days per week. When the non-emergency or non-urgent services of a specialist or acute care hospital are needed for the Centers' patients, as determined by the CRNPs at the Centers, the CRNPs will refer their patients to an appropriate physician or hospital based on the needs and wishes of the patient.

d. The Centers shall ensure that the CRNPs providing services at the Centers are appropriately licensed and qualified to practice as CRNPs in accordance with the laws of the commonwealth of Pennsylvania, including ongoing recertification, and will provide evidence thereof to DVCH upon request.

e. The Board of Pharmacy has determined that a physician's name currently must accompany each prescription. Therefore, the collaborating physician's name will be used when prescriptions are phoned into a pharmacy. Medications and other therapeutic measures are prescribed according to accepted protocols and community standards and in accordance with state and federal law.

4. **Compensation Issues.** The Centers will pay CH $100 per week for adult services and actually provided under this Agreement. No later than sixty (60) days before the end of each one-year term, either party may request to meet to review operations under the Agreement and to discuss the compensation payable for the subsequent year. Any change in compensation payable must be in writing and shall be incorporated into this Agreement.

5. **Insurance**

a. Throughout the term of this Agreement, the Centers and/or individual CRNPs shall maintain in effect the following:

   1. Appropriate professional liability insurance, in amounts consistent with applicable state law, to provide coverage for the CRNPs at the Centers in the performance of services at the Centers.

   2. Comprehensive general liability and employer's liability insurance with appropriate limits. The Centers will provide evidence of such insurance coverage to CH upon request.

b. Throughout the term of this Agreement, CH shall maintain in effect the following:

   1. Appropriate professional liability insurance, in amounts consistent with applicable state law, to provide coverage for its physicians in the performance of services pursuant to this Agreement.

   2. Comprehensive general liability and employer's liability insurance with appropriate limits. CH will provide evidence of such insurance coverage to the Centers upon request.

6. Indemnification:

a. The Centers and RHD shall indemnify and hold harmless CH, including, without limitation, CH agents, directors, officers, employees, other affiliated physicians, invitees, or guests, and any of CH's other contractors, from and against all claims, losses, costs, damages, and expenses (including, reasonable attorney's fees), relating to injury or death of any person or damage to real or personal property to the extent the above results from or arises in connection with the following:

    1. Any breach by the Centers of any provision of this Agreement.

    2. The negligent provision of medical services by the CRNPs at the Centers or failure to take certain action in connection with the provision of medical services including, without limitation, any negligence in failing to seek advice of a physician or to facilitate necessary transfer to an acute care hospital.

    3. Any other negligent act or omission by CH agents, directors, officers, employees, invitees, or guests, or any other parties involved in the performance of services under this Agreement.

7. Administrative and Miscellaneous Provisions:

a. **Independent Contractor Status.** In performing any or all services, and meeting any or all obligations provided for in this Agreement, CH shall at all times and for all purposes be and remain an independent contractor; and in no case and under no circumstances shall CH, or any of CH's employees, including, but not limited to, those employees who actually perform any services under this Agreement, be considered or otherwise be deemed to be employees of the Centers for any purpose whatsoever. Accordingly, neither the persons providing services pursuant to this Agreement not CH will receive or become entitled to any of the compensations or other employment-related benefits of any nature whatsoever including, but not limited to, workers compensation coverage, disability compensation or insurance, vacation, sick leave, life insurance, pension plan or benefits, or profit-sharing benefits, which employees of the Centers receive.

b. **Maintenance of Separate Identities and Control.** This Agreement shall not constitute, nor shall it be deemed or construed to be, a partnership, joint venture, or any other kind of entity of any nature whatsoever (whether juridical or otherwise) under the joint ownership or control of all or any of the parties of this Agreement. All parties to this Agreement shall remain separate and distinct entities and each shall continue to conduct business and affairs under the control of its own officers and board of directors, board of trustees, or other governing body, as the case may be, with such board of directors, board of trustees, or other governing body remaining solely responsible in all respects of the management conduct of the business and affairs of its institution. No party to this Agreement shall use the name or identity of any other party hereto for any purpose in any advertising, public relations communications, or other public communications without the prior written authorization of the party named or identified.

c. **Nondiscrimination.** Both parties agree that in the performance of this Agreement, there will be no discrimination against any patient, employee, or their person, on account of race, color, sex, sexual preference, religious creed, ancestry, age, handicap, or national origin. Such discrimination shall be cause for termination of this Agreement.

d. **Waiver of Breach.** The waiver of a breach of any of the terms hereof or any default hereunder shall not be deemed a waiver of any subsequent breach or default, whether of the same or similar nature, and shall not in any way affect the other terms hereof. No waiver shall be valid or binding unless in writing and signed by the parties.

e. **Modification.** No change or modification of this Agreement shall be valid unless it is in writing and signed by the parties hereto. Neither party shall assign its rights and obligations under this Agreement without the written consent of the other party; provided, however, CH shall have the right to assign this Agreement to any entity or institution controlled by, or under common control with CH shall have the right to assign this Agreement to another entity or institution under either their control.

f. **Governing Law.** This Agreement is made under, and shall be construed and enforced in accordance with, the laws of the Commonwealth of Pennsylvania.

g. **Integrated Agreement.** The parties agree that this Agreement constitutes the entire agreement between them with respect to the subject matter hereof and the transactions contemplated hereby, and supersedes all prior discussions, negotiations, and any preliminary, oral or written agreements, including all prior agreements with respect to the subject matter thereof.

APPENDIX K

Sample Nurse Practitioner–Collaborative Physician Practice Agreement

This agreement is designed to satisfy the minimum requirements of the Pennsylvania State Board of Regulations.

I. Parties to the Agreement

THIS AGREEMENT between _____, C.R.N.P., Certification number UP 000229-B (Certified Registered Nurse Practitioner) and _____, License Number MD 040618-E (Collaborating Physician) delineates the details of the collaborative arrangement between them with respect to the care of CRNP patients. The substitute physicians who will provide collaboration and direction for up to 30 days if the collaborating physician is unavailable is _____, MD 063140-L.

II. Area of Practice

The CRNP is certified in Family Practice.

III. Prescribing and Dispensing

This agreement authorizes the CRNP to prescribe and dispense drugs from the following categories:

(1) Antihistamines.
(2) Anti-infective agents.
(3) Antineoplastic agents, unclassified therapeutic agents, devices, and pharmaceutical aids if originally prescribed by the collaborating physician and approved by the collaborating physician for ongoing therapy.
(4) Autonomic drugs.
(5) Blood formation, coagulation and anticoagulation drugs, and thrombolytic and antithrombolytic agents.
(6) Cardiovascular drugs.
(7) Central nervous system agents, except that the following drugs are excluded from this category: general anesthetics and monoamine oxidase inhibitors.
(8) Contraceptives including foams and devices.
(9) Diagnostic agents.
(10) Disinfectants for agents used on objects other than skin.
(11) Electrolytic, caloric, and water balance.
(12) Enzymes.
(13) Antitussive, expectorants, and mucolytic agents.
(14) Gastrointestinal drugs.
(15) Anti-inflammatory medications.
(16) Local anesthetics.
(17) Eye, ear, nose, and throat preparations.
(18) Serums, toxoids, vaccines.
(19) Skin and mucous membrane agents.
(20) Smooth muscle relaxants.
(21) Vitamins.
(22) Hormones and synthetic substitutes.

IV. Prescription of Schedule II Substances

The CRNP may prescribe a Schedule II Controlled Substance for up to 72 hours when the CRNP and the Collaborating Physician have agreed that such prescription is in the best interest of the patient. Conditions include acute pain unrelieved by non-narcotic substances and when other appropriate medications were determined to be ineffective.

V. Professional Liability

The Professional Liability Insurance for the Nurse Practitioner is provided via the Federal Tort Claim Act. The amount of liability is one million dollars for each claim and three million dollars for aggregate occurrence.

VI. Attestation

The Physician attests that he/she has knowledge and experience with the drugs referred to in this agreement.

VII. Nature and Circumstance of the Collaboration

The Physician will see the patient in any of the following situations:

1. When in consultation or review, he/she decides it is necessary to do so.

2. When the CRNP decides it is outside his/her scope or experience.

Note: The Physician may recommend that another physician or specialist see the patient.

The emergency plan may be implemented in one or all of its parts.

VIII. Authorization

This agreement is valid as of the date signed by both parties. Notwithstanding the foregoing, the Agreement shall terminate if and when (i) the Physician is no longer licensed to practice medicine in Pennsylvania, (ii) the Physician dies or becomes disabled, (iii) the CRNP dies or becomes disabled, or has terminated employment with Resources for Human Development, Inc., or (iv) the parties mutually agree. This agreement will be reevaluated thirty days prior to the end of this agreement.

Nurse Practitioner: _____
Date: _____

Physician: _____
Date: _____

APPENDIX L

Sample Job Descriptions

THE FAMILY PRACTICE & COUNSELING
NETWORK EXECUTIVE DIRECTOR JOB
DESCRIPTION

JOB TITLE: NETWORK EXECUTIVE DIRECTOR

PRIMARY FUNCTION:
Upholds the mission and beliefs of the organization by assuring the delivery of evidenced-based primary care, behavioral health, oral health and enabling services to underserved people and by assuring fiscal stability, cost-effective care, and a high degree of staff and patient satisfaction.

QUALIFICATIONS:
RN License, minimum of a Master's Degree in Nursing or related health or management field. Minimum of two years experience in administration and work with low-income people.

SCOPE OF WORK RESPONSIBILITIES:

- Facilitates dialogue and communication in order to fulfill goals.
- Works with Health Center Advisory Board to monitor development and implementation of services responsive to the community.
- Assures that staff are hired from the community whenever possible.
- Conducts regular meetings with assigned "point person" and other corporate office staff as needed concerning significant health center issues such as plans for expansion, physical plant issues, program licenses, or significant employee problems.
- Fosters and maintains partnerships with the National Nursing Centers Consortium, Family Planning Council, Health Federation of Philadelphia, Primary Care Forum of Pennsylvania, Physicians for Social Responsibility and others to provide services responsive to the community.
- Assures that data such as UDS, federal and private grants, and interim reports are collected and reported in a timely manner.
- Works closely with fiscal director to monitor budget and productivity to assure sound financial operations.
- Sets budget with fiscal director and senior managers.
- Sets course for health center expansion to new sites and new programs in collaboration with senior leaders, RHD, and advisory board.
- Hires and directly supervises senior leadership team members, dental directors, and Information Technology Project director.
- Facilitates senior leadership team meetings once a month.
- Meets regularly with all senior leaders: works collaboratively with them to assure efficient and smooth operation of each department, assure that they have the tools and skills to carry out their work, assists in planning and problem solving.
- Conducts periodic performance appraisals of all direct reports.
- Obtains continuing education and management training to uphold regulations of managed care organizations, compliance with state, federal, and local requirements, and to grow as a responsible and dynamic leader.

PHYSICAL DEMANDS: Not Applicable

WORKING CONDITIONS: Normal

HAZARDS: Not Applicable

REPORTS TO: RHD and Health Center Advisory Board

_____

Supervisor's Signature

_____

Employee Signature

EFFECTIVE DATE: _____

JOB TITLE: DIRECTOR OF PRIMARY CARE SERVICES

Performance Evaluation:

MINIMUM QUALIFICATIONS:

- Current Pennsylvania state RN license
- Current Pennsylvania CRNP license
- Master's Degree in Nursing or a Management field

MINIMUM EXPERIENCE REQUIRED: Two years experience in management and work with low income people.

PRIMARY FUNCTION: Upholds the mission of the organization by assuring the delivery of primary care that is evidenced-based, satisfying to patients, and cost-effective; promotes a fiscally sound organization.

SCOPE OF WORK RESPONSIBILITIES:

Quality of Care:

- Facilitates dialog and communication in order to fulfill goals.
- Provides evidence-based primary care directly to patients carrying out all responsibilities as outlined in the job description of CRNP, including adherence to Clinical Practice Guidelines and Productivity Standards
- Responsible for hire, orientation, evaluation, and termination of all Nurse Practitioner and RN staff.
- Responsible for Nurse Practitioner office coverage and on-call scheduling.
- Assures the dissemination of clinical practice information to Nurse Practitioners and Medical Assistants.
- Acts as liaison and partner to Operations Director concerning OSHA and other governing regulations relative to Primary Care services.
- Performance Improvement: assures that primary care is monitored for adherence to Clinical Standards and addresses deficits.
- Assures the oversight of medication supplies.

- Acts as a resource to the Eleventh Street Director regarding the management of primary care operations at this site and meets at regular intervals
- Creates and oversees contractual relationships with collaborating physicians

*The PCD may assume the position of Primary Care Coordinator at one of the sites and if so, will fulfill the functions associated with this position.

Administrative:

- Serves as a member of the Senior Leadership Team
- Assures that the centers uphold requirements and contracts of partnered organizations such as The Family Planning Council, Reach Out and Read, Health Federation, the National Nursing Centers Consortium
- Collaborates with Network Executive Director in relation to fostering new partnerships with organizations that will result FPCN growth and services for new patients.

Supervision of Staff:

- Direct supervision of all NP Primary Care Coordinators and indirect supervision of RNs and CRNPs. Informally provides specific and concrete feedback on performance at least quarterly, performs formal review annually.
- Assigns Primary Care Coordinator to each site and delegates responsibilities as outlined in job description.

Fiscal Soundness:

- Sets productivity standards in collaboration with Network Executive Director.
- Interfaces with administrative staff concerning the creation and dissemination of Nurse Practitioner productivity reports at least quarterly, addresses deficits.

_____

Network Executive Director Signature

_____

Date

_____

Primary Care Director Signature

_____

Date

EFFECTIVE DATE: _____

JOB TITLE: CHIEF FINANCIAL DIRECTOR

MINIMUM QUALIFICATIONS: Bachelors Degree

MINIMUM EXPERIENCE REQUIRED:

- 10 years working in financial positions of increasing responsibility.
- 3 years in a management position.

PRIMARY FUNCTION:

Upholds the mission of the organization by assuming responsibility for all fiscal activities for the Family Practice and Counseling Network and assuring the fiscal soundness of the Network.

SCOPE OF WORK RESPONSIBILITIES:

- Facilitates dialogue and communication in order to fulfill goals.
- Provides advice and consultation on fiscal decisions to the Network Executive director and all members of the senior leadership team.
- Provides advice and financial forecasting on the feasibility of adding services.
- Prepares budgets for general operations and all grants.
- Meets with all department heads to prepare department budgets.
- Prepares Medicare and Medical assistance costs reports using a consultant as needed.
- Assumes responsibility for the completion and integrity of the UDS report.
- Assures that financial systems and staff are in place at all sites and that financial information and data are flowing between sites as required for Network fiscal operations.
- Coordinates relations with managed care organizations and third-party payer.

- Coordinates the fiscal, administrative, and contractual relationship between the FPCN/RHD and Drexel University.
- Maintains compliance with regulatory agencies as needed.
- Coordinates the daily execution of accurate and timely fiscal data entry, charge generation, billing, and collections performed by Fiscal Department employees.
- Provides monthly accounting reports and maintains accurate and reconciled balances for all Receivable Accounts with the corporate office.
- Authorizes and oversees the processing of all expenditures and maintains accurate and reconciled balances for all payable accounts with the corporate office.
- Oversees and authorizes payroll submissions to the corporate office.
- Assures the credentialing of all provider staff.
- Communicates with Network Executive director regarding anything out of the ordinary regarding finances.
- Serves as a member of the senior leadership team.

PHYSICAL DEMANDS: Not Applicable

WORKING CONDITIONS: Normal

HAZARDS: Not Applicable

REPORTS TO: Network Executive Director

_____

Supervisor's Signature

_____

Employee Signature

EFFECTIVE DATE: _____

JOB TITLE: OPERATIONS DIRECTOR

MINIMUM QUALIFICATIONS: Bachelors Degree

MINIMUM EXPERIENCE REQUIRED: 3 years experience in Management/Operations.

PRIMARY FUNCTION:

Upholds the mission and beliefs of the organization by working to assure that health care at the centers is affordable, accessible, and highly satisfying to patients, and by supporting the fiscal soundness of the Network.

SCOPE OF WORK RESPONSIBILITIES:

- Facilitates dialogue and communication in order to fulfill goals.
- Compiles statistical reports pertaining to CQI initiatives and health disparity analyses.
- Works with Network Executive Director on public relations and media activity.
- Sets up systems to solicit patient comments, satisfaction, tabulates results, and submits outcomes to CQI and appropriate supervisor.
- Arranges contracts, leases, and purchase of all major non-computer equipment such as fax, phone, and copiers in collaboration with Chief Financial Director.
- Oversees tickler for review of Personnel policies and procedures by senior leadership team.
- Oversees establishment and implementation of front desk operational procedures.
- Assures front desk compliance with any billing/financial procedures set by Chief Financial director.
- Oversees and maintains efficient patient flow.
- Facilitates all staff fun and team-building activities.
- Assures that outreach, transportation, and social services are provided to all eligible patients in a manner that is effective and satisfying to patients.
- Assures that health center physical spaces ar functional, clean and attractive.
- Oversees site renovations and relocations.
- Assures that administrative and clerical work necessary to support the Network and senior leaders is completed in an accurate and timely manner.
- Makes decisions that are specific to her department.
- Serves as a member of the senior leadership team.
- Direct supervises Fiscal Staff
- Direct supervision of Network Administrator

ADMINISTRATIVE RESPONSIBILITIES

- Oversee the Electronic Practice Management database operations.
- Oversee maintenance of all personnel files and related tracking systems.
- Oversee and authorize payroll submissions to Corporate office.
- Oversee purchasing and maintenance of program equipment and computers.
- Coordinate the maintenance of capital inventories for corporate office.
- Serves on the Senior Management Team.

PHYSICAL DEMANDS: None

WORKING CONDITIONS: Normal

HAZARDS: May be exposed to communicable disease.

SUPERVISORY RESPONSIBILITIES:

Direct supervision of site operations managers and administrative director.

REPORTS TO: Network Executive Director

_____

Supervisor's Signature

_____

Employee Signature

EFFECTIVE DATE: _____

JOB TITLE: DIRECTOR OF BEHAVIORAL HEALTH SERVICES

MINIMUM QUALIFICATIONS:

- An earned Master's Degree in a mental health field with a primary course of study in provision of therapy and counseling services, or equivalent training post-degree.
- Current license to practice in Pennsylvania.
- Good interpersonal skills and the ability to supervise, work independently, and as part of a team.
- Competency in working with individuals, families, couples, and groups with mental health problems, substance abuse problems and/or the dually diagnosed.
- Ability to maintain charts and provide reports as needed.
- Required updated training on mental health and substance abuse.
- Ability to utilize and follow all mental health and drug and alcohol licensing requirements of the state, insurance companies, and other funding sources.

MINIMUM EXPERIENCE REQUIRED:

Five (5) years experience as a therapist and/or clinical manager (may include student practicum experience if placement was full-time, and therapist received individual supervision from a licensed practitioner at least an hour a week).

PRIMARY FUNCTION:

Upholds the health center mission by assuring the delivery of high quality behavioral health services that receive a high degree of consumer satisfaction; assures the fiscal soundness of the organization.

SCOPE OF RESPONSIBILITIES AND TASKS:

I   Program Responsibilities
- A. Develop and implement programs and services in response to community need.
- B. Supervise and monitor job performance of Behavioral Health staff.
  1. Review charts for quality assurance
  2. Document supervisory sessions
  3. Prepare employee evaluations
- C. Initiate, coordinate, and monitor linkages to other providers and community organizations.
- D. Supervise and review all aspects of the Behavioral Health Program.
- E. Function as member of Health Center Senior Management Team.
- F. Meet jointly with Primary Care Provider team and Behavioral Health team at least five times a year.

II   Psychotherapy
- A. Conduct a minimum of 10 hours per week (for FT employee) of individual, couples, family, and/or group therapy.
- B. Manage the client load of all therapists with goal of maximizing insurance reimbursements.

III   Charting
- A. Complete all charting as needed and required by contracted funding sources including: intakes, psychosocial assessments, treatment plans, progress notes, service logs, and maintenance of psychiatric charting.
- B. Responsible for overseeing the charting of all therapists, student interns, and psychiatrists.

IV   Supervision
- A. Participate in supervision with the Executive Director monthly, or as needed.
- B. Participate in clinical supervision as needed and appropriate to level of training, with a Health Center approved supervisor.

V   Crisis Intervention
- A. Be immediately available to the Health Center staff during working hours in the event of a psychiatric emergency.
- B. Participate as a member of the Health Center Management Team in the event of any other kind of emergency.
- C. Monitor and participate in on-call rotation for mental health emergencies outside working hours.

VI   Coordination of Care
- A. Coordinate care of clients with the psychiatrist and the Health Center medical staff.
- B. Refer clients to other levels of care or other services as needed.

VII   Continued Education
Maintain competencies in mental health and substance abuse as required by licensing.

VIII   Member of Health Center's Multi-disciplinary Team
Attend Case Conferences and primary care/behavioral health integration meetings as scheduled.

IX Fiscal Viability
    A.   Set productivity standards with ED.
    B.   Monitor productivity, provide feedback to clinicians, and address deficits as indicated.

PHYSICAL DEMANDS: N/A

WORKING CONDITIONS: Normal

HAZARDS: N/A

REPORTS TO: Executive Director

_____
Supervisor's Signature

_____
Employee Signature

EFFECTIVE DATE: _____

JOB TITLE: THERAPIST

MINIMUM QUALIFICATIONS:

- One of the following:
  - An earned masters in social work or related field, with a minimum of 2 years experience as a therapist and a current license to practice in Pennsylvania.
  - An earned masters in psychology, with a minimum of 2 years experience as a therapist and a current license to practice in Pennsylvania.
  - An earned masters in psychology, with a minimum of 2 years experience as a therapist and currently working toward a doctoral degree in an applied mental health field.

- Good interpersonal skills and the ability to work independently and as a member of a team.
- Competency in working with individuals, families, couples, and groups with mental health problems, substance abuse problems, and/or the dually diagnosed.
- Good clinical writing skills and the ability to maintain client charts and provide reports as needed.
- Required updated training on mental health and substance abuse.
- Ability to utilize and follow all mental health and drug and alcohol licensing requirements of the state, insurance companies, and other funding sources.

PRIMARY FUNCTION:

Upholds the health center mission by assuring the delivery of high-quality behavioral health services that receive a high degree of consumer satisfaction; assures the fiscal soundness of the organization by meeting productivity standards.

PRIMARY RESPONSIBILITIES AND TASKS:

- **Psychotherapy**—Conduct a minimum of 17 hours (if full-time) of individual, couples, and/or family therapy a week, and groups as needed.
- **Charting**—Complete all charting as needed and required by contracted funding sources: including intakes, psychosocial assessments, treatment plans, progress notes, service logs, discharge planning, and maintenance of psychiatric charting.
- **Clinical Supervision**—Participate in supervision with designated Clinical Supervisor weekly. Participate in team meetings, case conferences, and interdisciplinary work groups as scheduled. Provide supervision to students/interns as needed, if appropriate to level of training and credentialing.
- **Crisis Intervention**—Be immediately available to the Family Practice & Counseling staff during working hours in the event of a psychiatric emergency. Participate as a member of the Family Practice & Counseling staff in the event of any other kind of emergency. Participate in regular rotation as on-call clinician after hours.
- **Coordination of Care**—Coordinate care of clients with the psychiatrist and the Family Practice & Counseling medical staff. Refer clients to other levels of care or other services as needed.
- **Continued Education**—Maintain competencies in mental health and substance abuse as required by licensing and funding bodies. Maintain current Pennsylvania license to practice OR maintain supervision that meets APA guidelines for student and/or postgraduate practicum, as appropriate to current level of training.
- **Member of Family Practice & Counseling's Multi-disciplinary Team**—Attend and participate in case conferences and primary care/behavioral health integration meetings as scheduled.

PHYSICAL DEMANDS: N/A

WORKING CONDITIONS: Normal

HAZARDS: N/A

REPORTS TO: Director of Behavioral Health Site Supervisor

_____
Supervisor's Signature

_____
Employee Signature

EFFECTIVE DATE: _____

Appendix M

Summary of HIPAA Requirements and Procedures

PRIVACY OF HEALTH INFORMATION POLICY

Definitions

Generally, terms used, but not otherwise defined, in these Policies shall have the same meaning given those terms in the Privacy Rule issued with respect to HIPAA (Health Insurance Portability and Accountability Act of 1996) and related laws. Otherwise, the following definitions pertain:

Business Associate means a person (including a corporate entity), other than an _____ employee, who participates in a function or activity involving the use or disclosure of protected health information (such as claims processing, information systems management, etc.) or provides legal, actuarial, accounting, consulting, data aggregation, management, administrative, accreditation, or financial services where the provision of the service may involve the use or disclosure of protected health information.

Consumer means a person who receives treatment by or through _____.

Health care means care, services, or supplies related to the physical, mental, or functional health of an individual that include preventive, diagnostic, therapeutic, rehabilitative, maintenance or palliative care, counseling, and assessment with respect to the physical, mental, or functional status or ability of an individual or which affects the structure or function of the individual's body. Most of our programs, under this definition, provide health care to our consumers.

Health care operations or **business operations**, as used in this policy and procedure document, means any _____ administrative activities to the extent that the activities are related to _____'s function as a health care provider, including: quality assessment and control, program evaluation, employment review of health care professionals, training of professionals, arranging for medical review, business planning and development, cost management, resolution of internal grievances, legal services, auditing and accounting services, fraud and abuse detection, and the like.

HIPAA Documentation means the single page documents, which are marked "HIPAA Documentation" and are appended to the Privacy Procedures, which document authorization, use, or disclosure of information or other matters as required by the Privacy Rule. HIPAA documentation shall be kept in a secure location for six (6) years from the date of its creation.

Payment means any activity undertaken by _____ for payment or reimbursement for the provision of health care, including billing, claims management, and efforts toward collection.

Personal Representative means a person who _____ will treat in the same manner as the consumer with respect to that consumer's health information in accord with state or federal law. Employees should check with their Unit Director before acting in response to any person other than the consumer with respect to that consumer's health information. Employees must keep in mind, especially here, that pertinent state and federal laws which affect the disclosure of health information (such as information under Federal Title X, information related to drug and alcohol rehabilitation, or information related to treatment for HIV/AIDS) are *NOT preempted*—generally meaning the more restrictive state or federal law controls. Not disclosing information to a person who could be a personal representative under HIPAA because another law prohibits it is more restrictive in this way.

Personal representatives include:

1. those who are authorized by state law to act on behalf of an adult or emancipated minor, such as those acting under a valid power of attorney or appointment as guardian;
2. with respect to minors, a parent, guardian, or other person acting *in loco parentis*, except that a minor has the authority to act as an individual if:
   a. the minor has consented to health service, no other consent is required under law, and the minor has not requested that another person be treated as the personal representative;
   b. the minor may lawfully obtain the health service without the consent of a parent, guardian, or person acting *in loco parentis*, and the minor, a court, or another person authorized by law consents to the service; or
   c. a parent, guardian, or person acting *in loco parentis* assents to an agreement of confidentiality between a RHD and the minor; and
3. with respect to deceased consumers, the next-of-kin if there is no established estate, or the estate administrator or executor if there is an established estate.

Notwithstanding whether a person meets the _____ definition of personal representative, an _____ employee must NOT disclose health information to any person other than the consumer if in sound professional judgment it is reasonable to believe that disclosure would endanger the consumer, another person, or it is otherwise not in the best interest of the consumer whose information is at issue. This is an important decision and should not be made without consultation with the Unit Director, a Corporate Assistant, or Associate Director.

Privacy Rule means the Standards for Privacy of Individually Identifiable Health Information at 45 CFR Part 160 and Part 164, Subparts A and E.

Protected Health Information means individually identifiable health information as more particularly described in the Privacy Rule and specifically excludes employment records held by _____ in its role as employer, such as workers compensation records.

Psychotherapy Notes means notes recorded (in any medium) by a mental health professional *documenting or analyzing the contents of conversations* during a private counseling session or a group, joint, or family counseling session and that are separated from the rest of the individuals' medical record. These do not include medication and prescription monitoring, counseling session start and stop times, modalities and frequencies of treatment, results of clinical tests, and any summary of the following items: diagnosis, functional status, treatment plan, symptoms, prognosis, and progress to date.

Treatment means the provision, coordination, or management of health care and related services to _____ consumers.

Unit means a division of _____, which operates under the direction of a Unit Director and may offer services to a class of consumers who are distinct from those served at other units in _____.

Policies

I. All _____ officers, employees, and agents shall preserve the integrity and the confidentiality of Protected Health Information pertaining to each consumer of _____'s services. This Protected Health Information shall be safeguarded to the highest degree possible in compliance with the requirements of the security rules and standards established under the Health Insurance Portability and Accountability Act of 1996 (HIPAA) and related regulations.

II. _____ shall publish and distribute to all Units a copy of these Policies and all subsequent amendments and shall direct that they be kept in an orderly manner in an accessible place for the information of the employees at the Unit.

III. _____ shall publish and distribute a Notice of Privacy Practices that informs the consumer in plain language about the uses and disclosures of Protected Health Information by _____, consumer rights in respect to uses and disclosures and limitations on _____'s use and disclosure of that information.

IV. _____ and its officers, employees, and agents will not use nor disclose an individual's Protected Health Information for any purpose not permitted. All such intended uses and disclosures will be listed on a Notice of Privacy Practices or, where not so disclosed, will not be used nor disclosed without the properly documented authorization of the consumer or his/her personal representative unless required by federal and/or state law.

V. _____ units may make additional policies meant to protect health information so long as those policies are not contrary to this _____ Privacy of Health Information Policy, are communicated to the unit's hub management in advance of the effective date of the unit's proposed policies, and are consistent with HIPAA and pertinent state and federal law.

VI. _____ shall take reasonable steps to limit the use and/or disclosure of, and requests for Protected Health Information to the minimum necessary to accomplish the intended purpose of the use, disclosure, or request.

VII. _____ shall implement reasonable administrative, technical, and physical safeguards to protect Protected Health Information from use or disclosure which violates the law.

VIII. _____ shall establish and maintain procedures to receive and address consumer complaints of unauthorized uses or disclosures of their Protected Health Information.

IX. _____ recognizes consumers' rights regarding their own Protected Health Information.

X. The consumer or the consumer's personal representative shall be granted access to their records subject to other pertinent law or the reasonable limitations related to the business processes of the organization unless, in the opinion of an appropriate medical professional, in accord with regulations, such access would be detrimental to the consumer.

XI. _____ recognizes that the consumer has the right to request amendment to the records to correct alleged inaccuracies. Such amendments shall be subject to law, professional ethics, and professional judgment and standards.

XII. _____ recognizes that the consumer has the right to request restrictions on the uses and disclosures of Protected Health Information and that the consumer is entitled to an accounting of disclosures of Protected Health Information for uses other than treatment, payment, and healthcare operations.

XIII. _____ shall establish contractual assurances from all business associates to which Protected Health Information is disclosed that the information will be used only for the purposes for which they were engaged, that they will safeguard the information from misuse, and that they will help the agency comply with its duties to provide consumers with access to health information about them and a history of certain disclosures.

XIV. _____ recognizes that neither HIPAA nor its related regulations preempt state and other federal laws except in such cases as these other laws may be contrary to HIPAA and related regulation; that is, the state or other federal law shall control unless it is impossible to abide by both simultaneously, in which case HIPAA and its related regulation shall control. Therefore and because _____ operates in more than several states, it shall keep abreast of the health information laws of these several states and shall operate lawfully in each of the states in which it does business.

XV. _____ shall create and maintain the office of Privacy Official, which shall be responsible for the development and implementation of the privacy policies and procedures. _____ shall also create and maintain the office of Contact Person, which shall be responsible for receiving complaints under the HIPAA laws and regulations. Theses offices may be assigned to employees with other assigned duties or to employees whose exclusive responsibility will be those related to these offices. RHD's Executive Director will make such assignments.

XVI. _____ shall provide adequate training related to the policies and procedures for compliance with the HIPAA privacy standards for all current employees and new hires. _____ will also provide updated training in a timely fashion to any employee whose functions are affected by a material change in the law, _____ policies, or _____ procedures. Training content and participation will be documented and retained by the Privacy Official.

XVII. All officers, employees, and agents of _____ shall comply with the standards set forth in this policy. Violation of this policy and unauthorized uses and/or disclosures of Protected Health Information are very serious offenses. Not only is policy violation grounds for disciplinary action, up to and including termination of employment, but violations related to unauthorized use and disclosure of Protected Health Information will be subject to severe sanctions. _____ shall make sure that each and every _____ employee is advised of this information.

XVIII. _____ shall make all reasonable efforts to lessen the harm caused by an improper use of disclosure of Protected Health Information by its workforce or by any business associate.

XIX. _____ shall maintain policies and procedures to implement HIPAA standards and regulations as these may change from time to time. RHD shall also maintain HIPAA Documentation for a period of exactly six (6) years from the date it is created.

XX. Ultimate responsibility for implementation and enforcement of these policies and procedures is properly placed with the Executive Director and the Privacy Official but all employees, especially assistant and associate directors, supervisors, and program coordinators, are responsible for enforcement. This policy is very important and employees who violate this policy, including by failure to properly enforce the policy and procedures, are subject to discipline.

APPENDIX N

Sample Performance Improvement Plan: Assessing Outcomes

Clinical Care Measures

Monitor #1

Perinatal Care

Indicator: Pregnant women presenting to any center in the network are referred for prenatal care and begin care within 1 week of discovering pregnancy.

Postpartum women enrolled as patients in the network receive a postpartum examination 6–8 weeks after delivery.

Postpartum women receive contraceptive management no later than 8 weeks after delivery.

Pregnant and postpartum women receive dental and oral screening during the prenatal and postpartum visits.

Pregnant and postpartum women are screened for depression.

Criteria: Medical records reflect referral and appointment date for beginning prenatal care within 1 week of discovering pregnancy.

Medical record reflects a postpartum examination no later than 8 weeks after pregnancy.

Medical records reflect contraceptive counseling and management to include permanent contraception, emergency contraceptive pills, and STD protection.

Medical records reflect dental and oral health screenings for all pregnant and postpartum patients.

Medical records reflect depression screening for all pregnant and postpartum women.

Expected Outcome: Increased access to prenatal care for all pregnant women presenting to any of the network

sites. Maintain continued access to free pregnancy testing on a walk-in basis.

Improved number of women receiving timely, comprehensive postpartum care.

Increased number of women receiving regular, reliable contraception postpartum.

Expanded number of women receiving preventive dental care during pregnancy and postpartum.

Improved identification and subsequent treatment of depression among pregnant and postpartum women.

Importance: There is documented disparity in infant mortality and low birth weight incidence when comparing patients served by the network to those in the city of Philadelphia as well as national figures.

Rationale: This indicator is high risk, high volume, and problem prone. Women in Philadelphia living in poverty are at a higher than average risk for poor prenatal care, low birth weight babies, and encountering barriers to access to high quality, respectful prenatal care.

Review Method: Chart review at defined intervals.

Sample Size: Review 20 of those patients with a positive pregnancy test or referral to the center's prenatal services during the review period. If patient volume is less than 20, 100% of the charts meeting criteria are reviewed.

Threshold: 100% of reviewed charts in compliance as outlined in criteria listed above.

Responsibility: Staff Nurse Practitioner

Clinical Care Measures
Monitor #2
Newborn/Infant Outcomes

Indicator:

- Newborn infants are seen at the network sites within 2 weeks of delivery.
- Newborn infants are seen at the network sites within the first month after birth.
- Infants are seen at the network sites at 2, 4, 6, 8, 10, and 12 months of age.
- Infants are assessed for growth and development at each well-baby visit.
- Infants are assessed for dental and oral health at each well-baby visit.
- Parent-infant interaction is assessed at each well-baby visit.
- Staff at each network site follows up with families for any and all missed well-baby appointments.

Criteria:

- Medical records reflect well-baby visit at 2 weeks, 1, 2, 4, 6, 8, 10, and 12 months of age.
- Medical records reflect that each well-baby visit includes assessments of growth and development, history of nutrition, sleep, elimination, and developmental milestones.
- Medical records reflect age-appropriate anticipatory guidance.
- Medical records reflect dental and oral health screenings for all infants during well-child exams.
- Medical records reflect assessment of parent-infant interaction and appropriate intervention where indicated.

- Medical records reflect lead studies on all infants enrolled in the network by 12 months of age.

Expected Outcome:

- Improved access to well-baby care.
- Improved assessment of infant growth and development.
- Improved discovery of failure to thrive and/or developmental delays.
- Improved early discovery of oral or dental health problems.
- Improve the identification and subsequent treatment of inadequate mother-infant interaction.

Importance: Infants living in the census tracks served by the network sites are at an increased risk for malnutrition, baby bottle tooth decay, developmental delay, and inadequate parenting secondary to maternal mental health problems and lack of education.

Rationale: Infants born to women living in the census tracks served by the network sites are more likely to be born to an adolescent and/or single parent who has limited financial, social, and emotional resources.

Review Method: Chart review done annually.

Sample Size: Review 25 infant charts that are representative of infants during the first year of life. If patient volume is less than 25, 100% of the charts meeting criteria are reviewed.

Threshold: 85% of reviewed charts in compliance as outlined in criteria.

Responsibility: Staff Nurse Practitioner

Clinical Care Measures
Monitor #3
Pediatric Growth and Development

Indicator:

- Children are scheduled at the network sites for well-child visits according to published guidelines from the APA.
- Children are assessed for growth and development at each well-child visit as per APA guidelines.
- Children receive vision and hearing screenings at each well-child visit as per APA guidelines.
- Children are assessed for dental and oral health at each well-child visit.
- Children receive Reach Out and Read information and books as per the Reach Out and Read Protocol.
- Cardiovascular risk assessment is performed and updated annually for each child receiving health supervision care at each network site.
- Children with chronic illness such as asthma or diabetes have a well-documented clear plan of care based on the latest evidence found in the literature.
- Parent-child interaction is assessed at each well-baby visit.
- Staff at each network site follows up with families for any and all missed health supervision appointments.

Criteria:

- Medical records reflect well-child visits at the recommended intervals.
- Medical records reflect that each well-baby visit includes assessments of growth and development, vision, hearing, hemoglobin, and a history of nutrition, sleep, elimination, and developmental milestones.
- Medical records reflect age-appropriate anticipatory guidance.
- Medical records reflect dental and oral health screenings for all children during health supervision visits.
- Medical records reflect assessment of parent-child interaction and appropriate intervention where indicated.
- Medical records reflect lead studies on all children enrolled in the network at 24 months of age.
- Medical records reflect appropriate referral for children with elevated blood lead levels.

- Medical records reflect a comprehensive management plan for all children with chronic illness such as diabetes or asthma.
- Medical records reflect developmental and mental health screening for all children receiving health supervision at the network primary care sites.

Expected Outcome:

- Improved access to well-child care.
- Improved assessment of child growth and development.
- Improved discovery of failure to thrive and/or developmental delay.
- Improved early discovery of oral or dental health problems.
- Improved discovery of children with elevated blood lead levels.
- Improved discovery and management of children with chronic illness.
- Improved discovery and treatment of children with mental illness.
- Improved identification and subsequent interventions to address inadequate mother-infant interaction.

Importance: Children living in the census tracks served by the network sites are at an increased risk for malnutrition, baby bottle tooth decay, developmental delay, chronic illness such as asthma, diabetes, or anemia, and inadequate parenting secondary to maternal mental health problems.

Rationale: Children born to women living in the census tracks served by the network sites are more likely to be born to an adolescent and/or single parent who has limited financial, social, and emotional resources.

Review Method: Chart review annually.

Sample Size: Review minimum of 20 pediatric charts representative of children from early, middle, and late childhood. If patient volume is less than 20, 100% of the charts meeting criteria are reviewed.

Threshold: 85% of reviewed charts in compliance as outlined in criteria.

Responsibility: Staff Nurse Practitioner.

Clinical Care Measures

Monitor #4

Pediatric and Adolescent Immunizations

Indicator: Pediatric and adolescent patients are offered immunizations as recommended by the American Academy of Pediatrics (AAP) and the Center for Disease Control (CDC).

Criteria: Medical records of pediatric patients reflect that immunizations were given at the recommended intervals, or at appropriate opportunities.

1. Immunizations given at the specified intervals.
2. Management plans established for parents who are non-compliant.
3. Documented evidence of guardian acceptance or refusal.

Expected Outcome: All children and adolescents are given immunizations at well-child checks or scheduled for immunizations at sick-child visits if the child is behind in his/her schedule, if and when appropriate.

Importance: Immunizations protect against specific preventable childhood diseases, and the morbidity and mortality associated with them.

Rationale: This indicator is high risk, high volume, and problem prone.

Review Method: Charts of children who are active users of the clinic are monitored on a semiannual basis for compliance with the criteria.

- Review "Pediatric Immunization Flow Sheets."
- Review "Patient Progress Notes."

Sample Size: At least 20 randomly selected charts. If patient volume is less than 20, 100% of charts meeting criteria are reviewed.

Threshold: 85% of pediatric and 95% of adolescent patients have age-appropriate immunizations.

Responsibility: Nurse Practitioners

Clinical Care Measures
Monitor #5
Adolescent Health Promotion and Preventive Services

Indicator: Adolescent patients receive ongoing periodic preventive health services.

Adolescent patients have dental screening and access to oral health services.

Adolescent patients are aware of community resources such as health fairs and Teen Awareness Day.

Adolescents with undiagnosed depression and primary mood disorders are identified by a nurse practitioner.

Sexually active adolescents receive reproductive health services such as contraceptive care and annual screening for chlamydia and other STDs. Couple/partner counseling sessions are encouraged.

Adolescents who are at-risk for drugs and alcohol are referred to appropriate clinicians, outreach staff, or community programs.

Adolescents receiving primary care receive the screening and counseling services recommended by the U.S. Preventive Task Force . . . sexual health, school performance, violence risk, depression/behavioral health assessment.

Criteria: Medical records on all adolescents reflect that preventive care is provided including all EPSDT screening, Denver Developmental Screening, immunizations, school progress appraisals, safety assessment, and education. Implement use of the revised Adolescent Health Maintenance Flow Sheet.

Medical records reflect referrals of at-risk adolescents to clinicians, outreach staff, or community programs.

Conduct outreach efforts in venues frequented by adolescents to explain health center services and enroll them in primary care.

Provide services to adolescents from Northern Home and Kirkbride Center (in-patient behavior health provider).

Sponsor and facilitate programs for teens including Teen Awareness Day, community health fairs, and Teen Parenting Group.

Medical records reflect assessment for oral health needs and referrals to contracted sites.

Expected Outcome: Increased number of adolescents receiving primary care at the health centers.

Increased preventive health services provided to adolescents.

Decreased violence, improved life skills, and self-esteem among adolescents.

Decreased use of tobacco, drugs, and alcohol among adolescents.

Decreased incidence of communicable diseases among sexually active adolescents.

Increased number of sexually active adolescents receive contraceptive and STD preventive services.

Increased rate of high-risk adolescent referrals to clinicians, outreach staff or community programs.

Improved identification of adolescents with depression and primary mood disorders.

Importance: Adolescents are less likely to use contraceptive methods due to impulsivity, lack of education, and other social/behavioral factors. Adolescents are also more likely to use drugs and alcohol secondary to low self-esteem and peer pressure. Nationally, it is reported that the incidence of chlamydia is at an epidemic proportion.

Rationale: These indicators are high risk, high volume, and problem prone.

Review Method: Medical and outreach records reflect the preventive and medical services rendered, including referrals. Review the Adolescent Health Maintenance Flow Sheet.

Sample Size: Review 20 charts of active users at each site.

Threshold: 100% compliance with criteria in 85% of the charts reviewed.

Responsibility: Nurse Practitioners, RNs, BH staff, Outreach Staff

Clinical Care Measures

Monitor #6

Adult Health Promotion and Preventive Services

Indicator: All patients 21+ years old receive screening for CV risks (both familial and environmental/habits) at routine physicals and periodic exams.

Criteria: CV screening are done at each visit by completing/reviewing the adult/adolescent flow sheet (smoking habits, family history of CAD prior to age 55, and other chronic illness co-morbidities) as well as through vital signs (checking blood pressure and pulse at each visit).

Laboratory studies are done on all patients at least annually to screen for CV disease (blood chemistries, fasting lipid panels for high-risk patients and all patients over 40 years of age).

Expected Outcome: 100% of adults have a CV risk assessment performed annually. All patients identified with hyperlipidemia or other cardiovascular diseases (hypertension, CHF) receive dietary and lifestyle modification teaching, counseling, medication, and referral to specialty providers as needed.

Importance: Patients in this population are at high risk for CVD due to tobacco abuse, high dietary fat intake, sedentary lifestyles, and heredity.

Rationale: This indicator is high risk, high volume, and problem prone.

Review Method: Charts of patients between 21 and 64 years of age are reviewed for compliance with criteria on an annual basis.

Sample Size: 25 charts of active adult users.

Threshold: 100% of adult patients are screened for CVD at least once annually based on criteria. 100% of patients identified with CVD will have annual fasting lipids, as well as dietary and lifestyle modification counseling.

Responsibility: Staff Nurse Practitioners and Primary Care Coordinators

Clinical Care Measures
Monitor #7
Geriatric Case Management

Indicator: Geriatric patients are provided quality care with appropriate case management services.

Criteria: Home visits to all new seniors as they move into the rebuilt Hope VI community across from the Falls site. Do in-home safety and health risk assessment, BP check, BS check, home medication review. Enroll interested seniors at the health center.

Documented assessment of seniors for depression, substance abuse, immunization status, chronic illness, safety, and needed services.

Link seniors to needed services such as meals on wheels, home health care, senior centers, and others.

Provide home visits to seniors as indicated.

Provide transportation and escorts to seniors for medical specialty care, dental, legal, housing, and other needed services.

Expected Outcome: Geriatric patients receive appropriate screening and care related to safety, chronic illness, immunizations, and mental health.

Importance: High-risk group. There are well-defined problems inherent and predictable in the geriatric population. Proactive approach in regards to preventative interventions and good health care has the potential to improve quality of life and is cost-effective in the long term.

Rationale: This indicator is high risk and problem prone.

Review Method: Chart audits via formal peer review process and review of outreach records.

Sample Size: 10–15 geriatric patients at each site.

Threshold: 100% of criteria met in specified % of records reviewed for each of the defined categories noted in the Network Health Care Plan.

Responsibility: PCCs, Outreach Coordinator, RNs

Clinical Care Measures
Monitor #8
Adult Immunizations

Indicator: All adult patients are given the opportunity, and encouraged where appropriate, to receive Td, Pneumococcal, Hepatitis, and Influenza vaccines according to CDC guidelines per age and risk.

Criteria: All geriatric patients will have evidence of a management plan for immunizations in their medical record as follows:

Patient education on the importance of these particular immunizations.

Td every 10 years.

Pneumococcal vaccine offered according to current CDC guidelines.

Influenza vaccine offered annually.

Hepatitis A and B vaccines offered based on risk or request for vaccine.

Chart documentation indicating acceptance or refusal.

Expected Outcome: Reduced risk of morbidity and mortality associated with these preventable diseases.

Importance: Patients served are high risk for injury and illness associated with socioeconomic and lifestyle factors inherent to this population.

Rationale: This indicator is high risk, high volume, and problem prone.

Review Method: Medical records of adult patients are reviewed for compliance with the criteria on a semi-annual basis.

- Review Adult Health Maintenance Flow Sheet
- Review Patient Progress Notes

Sample Size: 20 charts of active users of the clinic. If patient volume is less than 20, 100% of charts meeting criteria are reviewed.

Threshold: 100% compliance with criteria in 85% of the charts reviewed.

Responsibility: Nurse Practitioners

Clinical Care Measures
Monitor #9
Patient Satisfaction

Indicator: Patient satisfaction surveys conducted at each site twice per year.

Criteria: How long patient waited for appointment.

Convenience of office location.

Getting through to the office by telephone.

Length of time waiting to be seen by provider.

Amount of time spent with provider.

Explanations and education.

The technical skills of all staff.

Patient information was treated confidentially.

The visit experience OVERALL.

Whether you would recommend this center to your family or friends.

Expected Outcome: 90% of patients surveyed will rate care as Good to Excellent.

Importance: Word-of-mouth referrals have traditionally been our most common source for new patient registrations. Maintaining high patient satisfaction thereby serves our mission of expanding access to health care services as well as ensuring our ongoing viability.

Rationale: This indicator has broad consequences, both actual and potential in nature.

Review Method: Surveys administered at each site twice a year in May and October. Surveys tabulated by the NNCC and reported to CQI, senior managers, and all staff.

Sample Size: 100 from each site—total 400.

Threshold: 100% of criteria met in 90% of those surveyed.

Responsibility: Senior management, CQI committee, PCCs, all FPCN staff

Clinical Care Measures
Monitor #10
Staff Satisfaction

Indicator: Determine baseline staff satisfaction and turnover rates at individual sites and network.

Criteria: Employees receive job description, orientation, and know work expectations.

Employees have the information, materials, and equipment to do the job.

Employees are doing what they do best every day.

Employees receive performance evaluations and feedback.

Employees receive recognition or praise within 7 days.

Employees feel cared about as persons.

Employees receive encouragement for growth and development.

Employees feel their opinion is valued.

Mission/purpose convey importance and value of employees.

Expected Outcome: Increased staff retention and decreased staff turnover.

Increased opportunities to celebrate staff.

Increased opportunities for staff growth and development.

Job satisfaction reflected in staff satisfaction surveys.

Importance: Consistent, competent, and content (happy) employees provide the best service and care for our patients. Good job orientation, annual performance evaluation, and regular constructive feedback are essential for growth and development. Feedback is a collaborative obligation and a commitment to promoting success.

Rationale: Integral to the organizational Mission

Review Method: Monitoring/review of personnel records, staff satisfaction surveys, staff turnover data, and exit interview documentation annually.

Sample Size: 100% of Network employees.

Threshold: 100% of criteria met in 90% of those surveyed.

100% of criteria met in 100% of personnel records reviewed.

Responsibility: Administrative Director, Senior Management Team, and Administrative Assistant

Clinical Care Measures

Monitor #11

Access and Utilization

Indicator: Expanded service capability creating increased access and availability of services to target population. Subsequent user numbers expected to increase accordingly.

Criteria: 400 additional patients in year 1,400 in year 2, and 400 in year 3, for a total number of users of 3,800 at end of the 3-year period.

Expected Outcome: Expanded service capacity and increased number of users according to projections.

Importance: Highly relevant to organizational viability and continued success in meeting the Network's Mission and Goals.

Rationale: Increased service capability facilitates means to provide services to a greater number of people in the target population.

Review Method: Monthly reports/statistics on productivity, number of patient visits, new and ongoing users.

Sample Size: N/A

Threshold: Productivity 90–100% of projections.

Responsibility: Management team

PERFORMANCE IMPROVEMENT METHODS
P.D.S.A. (Plan, Do, Study, Act)

The Performance Improvement process is a continuous one. The end point in one area or study becomes the beginning point for the next cycle or study. The process we use has four parts known as 1) Plan, 2) Do, 3) Study, 4) Act.

PLAN: Based on the plan, identify an opportunity for improvement. Using statistical tools or some other analytical tool such as diagramming, force field analysis, etc., study the situation so that there is sufficient information available to form an opinion about how to improve the situation. Planning frequently takes the greatest amount of time of any of the steps because it is important that we understand enough about the problem or opportunity to be able to make a reasonable judgment about how to proceed as an organization. It is also important that we not succumb to "paralysis by analysis," that is, spend so much time with studying the detail of the problem that we never get around to attempting to actually do anything about it.

DO: Once a plan of action has been decided upon, assign responsibility for the task or tasks. It is extremely important that each element of the plan of action has a person individually responsible for the their part. Accountability is critical to ensuring that the plan of action is accomplished. Please remember that it is OK to fail. It is not OK to not try to make things work.

STUDY: This is the feedback of the process. Measurement and analysis through the use of statistical tools are used to make fact-based decisions about whether the plan of improvement actually did what was expected. Determine whether some aspects of the plan worked better than others. Look at ways to improve on the plan and continue "tweaking" the plan until the desired result is achieved.

ACT: Implement the change and decide how to hold the gains made in the process. Review the results of your activities to date on the issues being worked. It is important to note at this point that some ideas or projects are better simply abandoned. If things don't work or show promise of working, say so and move on to the next opportunity. Credibility in the PDSA process is important and must be maintained.

The cycle of PDSA is particularly important in looking at standardized processes such as making an appointment, generating a bill, or looking at protocols in clinical medicine. In each case the process followed has the same basic elements. This process can be used as easily by groups as by individuals and is the basis for our approach to continuous performance improvement.

References

Adams, C. M. (2002, January 8). Building credibility with grantmakers. *CharityChannel LLC, 1*(15).

Aydelotte, M. K., Barger, S. E., Branstetter, E., Fehring, R. J., Lindgren, K., et al. (1987). *The nursing center: Concept and design.* Kansas City, MO: American Nurses' Association.

Barger, S. E. (1995). Establishing a nursing center: Learning from the literature and the experiences of others. *Journal of Professional Nursing, 11*(4), 203–212.

Brush, B. L., & Capezuti, E. A. (1997). Professional autonomy: Essential for nurse practitioner survival in the 21st century. *Journal of the American Academy of Nurse Practitioners, 9*(6), 265–270.

Buppert, C. (1999). *Nurse practitioner's business practice and legal guide.* Gaithersburg, MD: Aspen.

Cherry, B., & Jacob, S. R. (2002). *Contemporary nursing: Issues, trends, & management* (2nd ed.). Philadelphia: Mosby.

Clemen-Stone, S., McGuire, S. L., & Eigsti, D. G. (2002). *Comprehensive community health nursing: Family, aggregate, & community practice* (6th ed.). Philadelphia: Mosby.

Elsberry, N., & Nelson, F. (1993). How to plan financial support for nursing centers. *Nursing & Health Care, 14*(8), 408–413.

Esposito, C. L. (2000). What's the point of malpractice insurance? *Nursing Spectrum, 12*(13), 6–7.

Fazzano, M. L. (2002). *Getting on the radar: How to approach family foundations.* Retrieved on October 18, 2002, from http://www.changingourworld.com/index.html

Free Clinic Foundation of America, Inc. (1998). *A free clinic: Starting out.* Roanoke, VA.

Frenn, M., Lundeen, S. P., Martin, K. S., Riesch, S. K., & Wilson, S. A. (1996). Symposium on nursing centers: Past, present and future. *Journal of Nursing Education, 35*(2), 54–62.

Glick, D. F., Hale, P. J., Kulbok, P. A., & Shettig, J. (1996). Community development theory: Planning a community nursing center. *Journal of Nursing Administration, 26*(7), 44–50.

Hansen-Turton, T., & Kinsey, K. (2001). The quest for self-sustainability: Nurse-managed health centers meeting the policy challenge. *Policy, Politics, & Nursing Practice, 2*(4), 304–309.

Hopkins, C. L. (1993). Establishing a nurse-managed center: A community approach. *Nurse Practitioner Forum, 4*(3), 165–170.

Jenkins, M., & Torrisi, D. (1997). Community partnership primary care case study: Abbottsford Community Health Center. *Nurse Practitioner Forum, 3*(1), 21–27.

Jenkins, M., & Torrisi, D. L. (1995). Marketing and management: Nurse practitioners, community nursing centers, and contracting for managed care. *Journal of the American Academy of Nurse Practitioners, 7*(3), 119–123.

Kerekes, J. J., Jenkins, M. L., & Torrisi, D. (1996). Nurse-managed primary care. *Nursing Management, 27*(2), 44–47.

King, E. (2002, November). NNCC Data Infrastructure Project. Presented at the National Nursing Centers Consortium bi-annual conference, Philadelphia, PA.

Kinsey, K. K., & Gerrity, P. (1997) Planning, implementing, and managing a community-based nursing center: Current challenges and future opportunities. *Handbook of Home Health Care Administration* (2nd ed.). New York: Aspen Publishers.

Lang, N. M., Sullivan-Marx, E. M., & Jenkins, M. (1996). Advanced practice nurses and success of organized delivery systems. *The American Journal of Managed Care, 2*(2), 129–135.

Lundeen, S. P. (1999). An alternative paradigm for promoting health in communities: The Lundeen Community Nursing Center Model. *Family & Community Health, 21*(4), 15–28.

Mundinger, M. O., Kane, R. L., Lenz, E. R., Totten, A. M., Tsai, W. Y., Cleary, P. D., et al. (2000). Primary care outcomes in patients treated by nurse practitioners or physicians: A randomized trial. *Journal of the American Medical Association, 283*(1), 59–68.

Riesch, S. K. (1992). Nursing centers: An analysis of the anecdotal literature. *Journal of Professional Nursing, 8*(1), 16–25.

Spitzer, R. (1997). The Vanderbilt experience. *Nursing Management, 28*(3), 38–40.

University Health Care Unit. (1991). *Workbook on establishing a nurse-managed health center*. New York: Center for Nursing Research and Clinical Practice.

Volunteers in Health Care. *Starting a free clinic basic starter kit*. Pawtucket, RI: Robert Wood Johnson Foundation.

Index

CPSIA information can be obtained at www.ICGtesting.com
Printed in the USA
266298BV00003B/5/P